Praise for *The Healthiest People on Earth*

"A fascinating and important book that I hope will inspire many more people to embrace optimal nutrition and improve their quality of life."

—T. COLIN CAMPBELL, PHD, coauthor of international bestseller *The China Study* and the *New York Times* bestseller *Whole*

"With humor and a rich family history, John Howard Weeks brings the basics of Blue Zone living into the new millennium—and right into your own kitchen. By showing how to take the steps to plant-sourced eating and healthy living with ease, along with a fresh 'Happy Home Remedy' punctuating every chapter, Weeks lays the groundwork for creating your own thriving Blue Zone—easily, and anywhere in the world."

—LANI MUELRATH, author of *The Mindful Vegan*, *The Plant-Based Journey*, and *Fit Quickies*

"A joyful romp through John Howard Weeks's life and discovery that to live energetically and healthily he needed to change what he chose. Choosing to live a vibrant life, he chose a plant-based diet. Choice is key. He demonstrates how anyone can do the same. In his lively conversational tone, Weeks tells how he fell from health and how he returned. Offering practical tips, remedies, and recipes, he also shines light into North America's only Blue Zone in which people live on average ten years longer than others."

—JEFF STANFORD, coauthor of *Dining at The Ravens*

"John Howard Weeks has written a book for people like me—who love life and want to live as long as possible. It's an accessible, practical guide for how to adopt optimal habits and enjoy the process. Easy to read, and easy to do!"

—PAMELA A. POPPER, PHD, ND, president of Wellness Forum Health

"I believe that everyone should want to live as healthy as possible for as long as possible. In a compassionate, honest, and articulate manner . . . sprinkled in with brilliant humor and candor . . . author John Howard Weeks presents in *The Healthiest People on Earth* a whole life lesson for us that will serve as a blueprint for reaching that goal."

—NICHOLAS R. CATALDO, author, educator, and San Bernardino County historian

"If you want to learn how to live a healthier lifestyle and perhaps live a little longer, this book will show you how. Thankfully, Weeks's gentle humor makes the whole prospect very easy to digest."

—JOHN PLESSEL, columnist for the *Southern California News Group* and food blogger for Dine 909

"There are many books talking about healthy eating but reading *The Healthiest People on Earth* really gives you convincing data that following a vegetarian diet really is better for you. John Howard Weeks has the uncanny ability to make the reading easy and engaging. I guess it's time for me to alter my diet! I encourage everyone to read this life enhancing book."

—ALLAN BORGEN, food critic and host of the PBS
television and radio show *Let's Dine Out*

"John Howard Weeks's latest book, *The Healthiest People on Earth*, is more than packed with information to create your own 'Blue Heaven on Earth' (a Blue Zone). It is a fascinating, easy, and fun read!"

—BILLIE J. RUBEN, natural health activist and 18-year cancer
survivor without surgery or chemotherapy

"Weeks nails it! This important work is the latest in a growing body of evidence that a plant-based diet is the path to longevity and quality of life. A must-read for all who want fewer doctor visits and lower medical bills."

—ROBERT S. PETERSON, MPH, former director of Public Health Education
at Castle Medical Center in Kailua, Hawaii

"This is an informative yet really enjoyable and honest book about living your life to the fullest. People who know me know I used to love to eat meat. But I became a 95% vegetarian over a year ago because I finally read *The China Study*, which John talks about in *The Healthiest People on Earth*. I wish that I had known the facts about eating well when I was growing up. I would have never eaten meat. This book shows how anyone can change."

—PHIL YEH, graphic artist, author, and creator of *The Winged Tiger*

"I have to admit that I'm not a big reader of diet instruction. However, having started in on this book I realized it was very different from the normal type. Firstly, Weeks's sense of humor soon spills over into what is, after all, a somewhat dry subject. Secondly, although it follows the dietary precepts of Seventh-day Adventists, there's not a trace of religion in it. For that I was glad as I've always been suspicious of congregations who believe the Deity is concerned with our food selections. No, *The Healthiest People on Earth* is simply a guide to how we can benefit from a diet that is almost certain to not only prolong our lives but to help us keep out of the doctor's office. Throughout the book, I kept feeling that this all made absolute sense and in fact, it is the right thing to do. What is also helpful, however, is a complete chapter on cheating, if you fall off the rails from time to time."

—Trevor Summons, columnist and author of *Trevor's Travels*,
Requital, *Transposition*, *McConnells*, and *A Charmed Life*

The Healthiest
People on Earth

The Healthiest People on Earth

Your Guide to Living 10 Years Longer with
Adventist Family Secrets and Plant-Based Recipes

JOHN HOWARD WEEKS

*The Great-Great-Grandson of Seventh-day Adventist
Founder Ellen G. White*

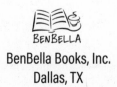

BenBella Books, Inc.
Dallas, TX

BenBella Books, Inc.
10440 N. Central Expressway, Suite 800 | Dallas, TX 75231
www.benbellabooks.com | Send feedback to feedback@benbellabooks.com

Printed in the United States of America
10 9 8 7 6 5 4 3 2 1

Library of Congress Cataloging-in-Publication Data
Names: Weeks, John Howard, 1949- author.
Title: The healthiest people on earth : your guide to living 10 years longer
    with Adventist family secrets and plant-based recipes / John Howard Weeks,
    the great-great-grandson of Seventh-day Adventist founder Ellen G. White.
Description: Dallas, TX : BenBella Books, Inc., [2018] | Includes
    bibliographical references and index.
Identifiers: LCCN 2017047920 (print) | LCCN 2017048798 (ebook) | ISBN
    9781946885227 (electronic) | ISBN 9781944648862 (paperback : alk. paper)
Subjects: LCSH: Longevity—Nutritional aspects. | Health—Religious
    Aspects—Seventh-day Adventists. | Medicine—Religious
    Aspects—Seventh-day Adventists. | Vegetarianism—Recipes.
Classification: LCC RA776.75 (ebook) | LCC RA776.75 .W444 2018 (print) | DDC
    613.2—dc23
LC record available at https://lccn.loc.gov/2017047920

Editing by Scott Calamar
Copyediting by Karen Levy
Proofreading by James Fraleigh and Jenny Bridges
Indexing by Debra Bowman
Text design and composition by Silver Feather Design
Front cover by Oceana Garceau
Full cover by Sarah Avinger
Printed by Lake Book Manufacturing

Distributed to the trade by Two Rivers Distribution, an Ingram brand
www.tworiversdistribution.com

I dedicate this book with love to my family—my brother Douglas Alan, his wife Richelle, and their daughters Elizabeth and Kate; my sister Carolyn Marie; my sister Donna Louise, her husband Blaine Simpkins, and their son John Douglas; my father and mother Howard Benjamin Weeks and Dorothy Mae White Weeks; my grandparents Herbert Clarence White and Anna Louise Johnson White; my great-grandparents William Clarence White and Ethel May Lacey White; and my great-great-grandparents James Springer White and Ellen Gould Harmon White.

This is not a book about religion.
It is a book about health and happiness.

There are more than 20 million Adventists
throughout the world, and they are remarkable for their longevity.

This book tells you how they do it, and how you can do it, too.

Contents

INTRODUCTION

Bad Tidings, Then Glad Tidings

HUMANS ARE FAT AND SICK. WE ARE FATTER AND SICKER THAN WE EVER HAVE been. And we are getting fatter and sicker all the time.

Americans are the worst, but people who live in other Western or Westernized nations aren't much better. Sadly, we're all in bad shape.

As a human myself, I am concerned for us.

We spend staggering amounts of money on health care, but we don't have better health to show for it. Heart disease, hypertension, stroke, cancer, osteoporosis, and diabetes are so rampant and on the rise in our part of the world that they are called "Western diseases."

Obesity is at the epidemic stage. About 70 percent of Americans are overweight, and more than half of those are obese, according to a report in the June 2015 issue of *JAMA Internal Medicine*, a publication of the Journal of the American Medical Association. American children, even infants, are so fat that they are coming down with "adult" diseases like diabetes. Experts worry that children of the future may not outlive their parents.

We eat fatty, greasy, sugary, salty food, and we eat far too much of it.

We are fattening ourselves at a rate that has made it necessary to widen doorways and manufacture larger, sturdier chairs. Commercial airliners must gas up with extra jet fuel to carry today's heavier passengers. Bigger hospital beds and operating tables are being built.

And bigger caskets.

Is there any defense against this deadly trend?

Yes, there is.

More and more studies are showing that good nutrition is miraculously more effective than drugs or surgeries in preventing and even curing disease. And, happily, we are blessed to live on a bountiful planet bursting forth with nutrition-rich fruits, vegetables, whole grains, and healthy proteins.

We have all the good things to eat and drink that will keep us healthy and bright-eyed. Why on Earth would we choose to eat and drink those few things that make us unhealthy and dull?

Yet, millions of us do.

I myself was among those millions. And I have no excuse.

I come from a long line of health crusaders, going back four generations. My great-great-grandmother, Ellen G. White, was founder and prophet of the health-smart Seventh-day Adventist church, and she preached diet and health reform throughout her long life (1827–1915). She pioneered and popularized vegetarianism in America and around the world. Her many books have appeared in so many languages that she is acknowledged as the most translated female author in history. For this and other reasons, she was named one of the "100 Most Significant Americans of All Time" in a Spring 2015 special edition of *Smithsonian* magazine.

Today, the Adventist church continues to teach and practice Ellen G. White's "whole person" concept of wellness that emphasizes health of body, mind, and spirit. The church has grown to become the world's twelfth largest, with a membership of more than 20 million. Its global outreach includes not only 70,000 churches located in more than 200 nations, but also more than 600 hospitals and other care centers.

Now, you might think that with my pedigree as a direct descendent of the founder of this church, I probably have been a total health nut my whole life. Right?

Wrong.

Alas, I strayed.

I rebelled against my family, my genes, my heritage, my destiny. I turned my back on the unique wisdom handed down to me by my ancestors. I made a million mistakes.

But over time I learned from each one of them.

Apparently, I had to give all the wrong choices a try before I understood how to make the right ones.

Overeating? Been there.

Smoking? Done that.

Drinking? Still working on that one, but making progress.

Slacking? Oh, yes, I went from physically fit as a young man to physically phhht as a grown man.

But then I turned things around. I decided it was time for a change, so I made one. I made lots of them. I became a health nut. Finally!

It took time. It took effort. On every level, I had to relearn and redeploy the lessons of my privileged youth to reform and reshape myself into the amazing specimen of manhood you see before you today. Oh, wait. I guess this isn't a picture book. (Whew!)

I'm going to tell you everything about how I did it and how you can do it, too. And you can trust what I say because I am battle-tested. I earned every one of my victories in hand-to-hand combat with that little devil of temptation that sits on my shoulder. You can win the battle with your little devil, too.

I'll show you how.

You'll be delighted to find out that the world's best diet is also the easiest, cheapest, least complicated, and most delicious. It will take lots of miserable pounds off your weary frame, and almost certainly will add lots of happy years to your life.

You'll be thrilled to learn that the world's best exercise is something that you already do every day. You just need to do a little bit more of it.

We're going to cheer up that irritable bowel of yours. You're going to want to sit down for that news!

Oh, we are going to accomplish a lot of things.

You're going to sleep more soundly than you have slept in a long, long time. And you'll have better dreams, too.

You're going to find out that sex can get better and better, not worse and worse, as you grow older. Oh, yes, we will be talking very frankly, very candidly, very intimately about sex. Lucky this isn't a picture book.

(You wish!)

We're going to talk about everything. Good muscles. Good bones. Good skin and more.

The cure for the common cold? Yep, that's in here, too.

There also are recipes for a lot of wonderful dishes that you are going to love.

Some of them go way back, more than a hundred years, to the time of my great-great-grandmother and the founding of Adventism. These recipes are printed here for the first time anywhere.

We're going to learn a lot together, you and I, and we also are going to have fun. We're going to laugh a lot, shout a lot, and wave our arms a lot as we go along.

There is no religion in this book. Not one bit of it anywhere. Yes, I know you may be worried, because I just told you that I come from a family that founded a church. But it's a church with a health message as well as a faith message, and health is all we are discussing here. No theology allowed.

I think you'll find that my lineage is interesting in ways that you will find worthwhile, because I have a lot of good family stories, and juicy family secrets, and even delicious family recipes to share that will surprise you!

I'm only in the middle of my own journey of discovery, and I am sure I have much more to learn, but I already have learned much. I've learned that, while no one is perfect, each one of us has the opportunity and the tools to be as optimally healthy as we possibly can be. And I mean healthy in that "whole person" way. Healthy in body, healthy in mind, and healthy in spirit.

That's pretty close to perfection in my book.

There I go, plugging my book!

It's because I want you to read it. I want you to join me on the quest for perfection. It's good to have company on an adventure this big. It's good to share an experience this important.

First, we must throw out the old maps, guides, and playbooks that most people use to seek their path through life. We have to play by new rules. We need to let go of a lot of cherished notions. We need to steal into the temple of old ideas and smash some idols.

The temple. Wow, there's a concept. You've heard the expression "the body is a temple"?

Well, in olden times, temples often were the scenes of barbaric sacrificial rites involving much butchering, bloodletting, and carnage.

Hopefully, this is not the sort of temple we mean when we talk about our bodies being temples.

Yet, millions of people act that way. They use their bodies as places of sacrifice. Yes, it's where they sacrifice their self-control, their judgment, their moderation, their good sense, their well-being, even their dignity.

Fortunately, it's possible to follow a better course. It's possible to achieve an ideal state of being. It's possible, in short, to be healthy.

Healthy in body, mind, and spirit.

Now, let me say it straight up front, I am not a doctor.

Thank heaven!

Doctors concentrate almost all of their attention on disease and damage. They use surgeries and drugs in costly, often futile repair attempts. In fact, that's what doctors are—repair specialists. As well-meaning as they may be, they make their living on sick people, not well people. They don't bother too much with nutrition and fitness, which are the vital keys to health that help prevent sickness in the first place. Doctors spend long years in medical school, but they spend little or no time learning about diet and exercise. It's just not part of the curriculum. Believe me, I know. My extended family includes many fine doctors, and I've heard all of their stories.

Doctor's offices and hospitals are where you go for intervention. Not prevention. Not protection.

Here's more bad news. If it's protection you want, there are many commercial and industrial forces arrayed against you.

Food companies want you to come back for more, so they load up their products with addicting sweeteners, chemical additives, and processed oils, fats, and grease.

The U.S. Department of Agriculture plays sidekick to the food companies. The USDA's crazy "nutrition guidelines" should be labeled "bad nutrition guidelines." You remember that old "food pyramid" of theirs, right? I had to laugh at that one. I couldn't help reflecting on the fact that pyramids were used to entomb the dead.

The health insurance companies, meanwhile, hope you'll feel sick and scared enough to buy their most expensive plans. They make money by betting that you'll bet against yourself.

The drug companies make enormous fortunes selling their dope to people who are sick and scared.

Hospitals make money by renting beds by the hour to people who are sick and scared.

Yes, there's a lot of money to be made from people who are sick and scared, and there are far too many millions of us who keep coughing it up.

Fortunately, I'm here with good news. We can stop this madness. We can battle back against these forces and win.

What's our strategy?

We stop being sick and scared.

That's all it takes.

I'm going to show you how easy it is.

BONUS: Throughout this book you will find news you can use to boost your health and well-being. To make extra sure of it, I am adding a special tip, each one called "A Happy Home Remedy," to the end of every chapter. There also is an entire chapter of additional "Happy

Home Remedies" later on, as you will see. Many of these tips are based on the collected lore handed down through generations of my own family. I hope you will find each one of them to be interesting and useful. Here's the first one.

A Happy Home Remedy That Reveals a Single Word You Can Use to Vastly Improve Your Diet

---

The U.S. Department of Agriculture finally has disavowed its notorious "food pyramid" after years of controversy. The icon, introduced in 1992, was intended to illustrate the correct combination of food groups in a healthy meal. Instead, what it depicted was a carbo-loaded calorie-swollen catastrophe.

Six food groups were featured, with grains (bread, cereal, rice, and pasta) comprising the entire foundation level, then fruits and vegetables sharing side-by-side smaller spots in the next level, then meat and dairy sharing smaller side-by-side spots in the next level, and finally "fats, oils & sweets" proudly occupying the little triangle on top.

A revised pyramid in 2005 was pared down to five food groups: grains, fruits, vegetables, meat, and dairy. The "fats, oils & sweets" were ditched. Next, the whole pyramid vanished, giving way in 2011 to MyPlate, a new icon that shows two plates. Fruits, vegetables, grains, and protein fill four spots on a large dinner plate, and dairy occupies a smaller plate on the side.

Better? Perhaps, but it definitely can be improved. For starters, let's add a single word to the "grains" category. Let's call it the "whole grains" group. That single word, "whole," is very important.

Always, always, always choose bread, cereal, rice, and pasta that is labeled "whole grain." This means that the grain is intact, in its natural state, and not processed and stripped of its essential nutrients. By observing this one word, you will be enjoying food that fuels your body with healthy carbohydrate energy, instead of food that fools your body with junk calories.

CHAPTER ONE

In the Zone

MY HOMETOWN, LOMA LINDA, LOCATED SIXTY MILES EAST OF LOS ANGELES in Southern California, is America's only entry on the short list of so-called Blue Zones, which are regions of Earth where people live measurably longer than average. Almost a decade longer, in fact.

Not coincidentally, Loma Linda is also a Seventh-day Adventist stronghold, where meat markets, liquor stores, and tobacco shops are not to be found in the downtown city center. Loma Linda is a key bastion of the denomination's worldwide health outreach. It is home to the famed Loma Linda University School of Medicine and LLU Medical Center, where health of body, mind, and spirit are taught and practiced. "To Make Man Whole" is the institution's motto. LLU operates some of the largest clinical programs in the nation and cares for 33,000 inpatients and 500,000 outpatients each year.

Loma Linda is a small city in terms of population (about 20,000) but it is huge in terms of health care resources. There actually are five separate but affiliated hospitals clustered within blocks of each other. In addition to the mothership, LLUMC, there is the LLU Children's Hospital, the LLU Heart and Surgical Hospital, the Jerry L. Pettis Memorial Veterans Medical Center, and Loma Linda University Medical Center East Campus (formerly Loma Linda Community Hospital).

Loma Linda's conglomerated health care services attract a worldwide clientele.

The city also is home to the Loma Linda Market, one of the nation's first health food stores, founded in 1936. And it is the birthplace of Loma Linda Foods, established in 1933, a pioneer manufacturer of plant-protein meat substitute products. Until its recent (October 2016) acquisition by Nashville-based Atlantic Natural Foods, Loma Linda Foods was a division of the Kellogg Company, founded in 1906 by W. K. Kellogg, who, with his physician brother John Harvey Kellogg, invented and perfected the recipe for corn flakes. The Kellogg brothers were Seventh-day Adventists.

Now, here's an oddity to consider. The Southern California city of San Bernardino is Loma Linda's immediate next-door neighbor to the north, but it is a totally different kind of place. It's home to the original "Berdoo" chapter of the Hells Angels motorcycle club, and it also is the birthplace of the fast-food industry. It's where the McDonald brothers, Richard and Maurice (Mac), revolutionized the restaurant business and the American diet when they converted their San Bernardino hamburger joint into a drive-in in 1948.

Their timing was perfect. World War II had ended and a new era of busy prosperity was at hand. American soldiers came home and many of them bought their first automobiles. A new car culture was about to be born. A new hurry-up attitude was taking hold.

The McDonald brothers streamlined their menu and offered "Speedee" service. They worked with local machinists to develop new devices that could whip up milkshakes right in the cup, dispense uniform dollops of ketchup and mustard, peel potatoes in mass quantities, and fry up hamburgers by the thousands, each one identical, in record time.

McDonald's was a sensational success, and other entrepreneurs took notice. For example, the fledgling founders of KFC, Carl's Jr., and Wendy's all made pilgrimages to San Bernardino to study the brothers and their methods. Another budding fast-food king, Ray Kroc, was so smitten that he bought franchise rights, and later the whole company, from the brothers.

Others who were impressed by the food revolution happening in San Bernardino included a couple of local boys. They were buddies, in fact, who had graduated from San Bernardino High School together, served in the war together, and returned home together. Marveling at the crowds they saw at McDonald's, they sought and received tutelage from the McDonald brothers. Then, in the early 1950s, they put their lessons into practice. Glen Bell opened a Mexican fast-food restaurant called Taco Tia, which became a popular regional chain that still exists. His friend Neal Baker invented the "Twin Kitchen" concept with hamburgers at one window and Mexican food at another window at his Baker's Burgers drive-ins, which also grew to become a popular local chain that is still in business.

Bell went on to popularize the fast-food hot dog, opening a restaurant he called Der Wienerschnitzel. Then he had an even bigger idea, so he sold Der Wienerschnitzel to one of his employees, John Galardi, and proceeded to start a new chain of Mexican fast-food restaurants named after himself, Taco Bell, which today is America's largest purveyor of its kind with about 6,000 outlets. Another Bell employee, Ed Hackbarth, started the Del Taco chain, now America's second-largest provider of Mexican fast food, with more than 500 drive-ins.

Meanwhile, Galardi turned Der Wienerschnitzel into America's largest fast-food hot dog chain with about 400 locations.

And, of course, McDonald's went on to become what today is the largest restaurant chain of any kind on Earth, the most prodigious supplier of fast food on the planet, feeding nearly 70 million people each day in more than 36,000 drive-ins located in 119 countries throughout the world.

Remember, ground zero for all of this is San Bernardino, right next to Loma Linda. It's a short hop from the site of the original McDonald's in midtown San Bernardino to the Loma Linda Market in the heart of Loma Linda.

Nutritionally speaking, this is a bizarre place in which to grow up, as I did. I always have enjoyed the comic irony of living in the X spot where the world capital of junk food butts up against the world capital of health food. In one corner, we find the meat chewers. In the other corner, we find the meat eschewers.

It's a wonder to me that there hasn't been war.

COMMANDER OF THE LOMA LINDA FORCES: "They're ramming the gates with an enormous log of summer sausage!"

COMMANDER OF THE SAN BERNARDINO FORCES, USING A BULL-HORN: "Surrender, or we'll start catapulting giant, squishy meatballs over the wall!"

COMMANDER OF THE LOMA LINDA FORCES, RALLYING THE TROOPS: "To your battle stations! Prepare to fire the cabbage cannons!"

To give each party its due, it must be acknowledged that junk food has trended much better, in terms of popularity, than health food. The culinary message coming out of San Bernardino has resonated with far more people than the one coming out of Loma Linda. San Bernardino has spawned, either directly or indirectly, most of the world's biggest fast-food chains. On the other hand, there is no chain of Loma Linda Markets. It hasn't gone global, like McDonald's has. There are far fewer people in the world eating veggie burgers than hamburgers today.

But Loma Linda is a Blue Zone, one of the very few places on Earth where people live longer, healthier lives than anyone else.

San Bernardino definitely is not a Blue Zone. Not even close. In fact, though the two cities sit side by side, they are a million miles apart, nutritionally speaking.

The Blue Zone research, backed by *National Geographic*, was reported first by author and researcher Dan Buettner in his best-selling book *The Blue Zones: Lessons for Living Longer from the People Who've Lived the Longest*, originally published in 2008 and then revised in a second edition published in 2012. Loma Linda is featured in a chapter titled "An American Blue Zone."

As the chapter points out, Seventh-day Adventists, who founded Loma Linda and still dominate its population, enjoy a strong community support system that fosters a convivial, equanimous, low-stress lifestyle. Generally speaking, they also eat a totally or mostly vegetarian diet, plus they shun tobacco, abstain from or limit their use of alcohol, and embrace the virtues of regular exercise and sound rest. Similar attributes are to be found in the world's four other Blue Zones: Okinawa Island in Japan, the Barbagia region of Sardinia in Italy, the Nicoya Peninsula of Costa Rica, and the Greek island of Ikaria.

Another best-selling book, *The Secrets of People Who Never Get Sick* (2010) by journalist and researcher Gene Stone, devotes its first chapter to the Blue Zones. The Blue Zone research is summarized in general terms, and the specific point is made, in discussing Loma Linda, that the Seventh-day Adventists are "the longest-living group of people in America."

Growing up in Loma Linda, I always knew it was a special place. A different place.

Meat was nowhere to be found. There were no restaurants that served it. There were no grocery stores that sold it. There were no meat smells in the air. You never sniffed a roast cooking in someone's kitchen. You never smelled steaks grilling on a backyard barbecue.

I think it was in 1967, when I was a high school senior at Loma Linda Academy, that a heathen café dared to open its doors in downtown Loma Linda and serve meat dishes. Believe me, it didn't last long. The community leadership rose up in wrath, accusing the restaurant of fraudulently representing itself in its permit application. It was a moot point, as it turned out, because the restaurant attracted no business at all. In fact, nervous citizens would cast fearful glances down that street and they would quicken their step if they had to walk that way. It was as if the Devil himself had opened up a diner.

To the best of my knowledge and recollection, that sort of terrible devilry never has been attempted since, to this very day.

Oh, to be sure, in recent years, as Loma Linda has grown and prospered and attracted increasingly diverse additions to its population, it has become a little more worldly. Flesh-food restaurants, fast-food drive-ins, and markets with butcher counters now can be found on the city's outskirts. But no such establishments can be found downtown, in the heart of the campus and business district. The Loma Linda Market, which possesses exclusive title there, is completely meat-free, as it always has been. You can't even buy a little bottle of Worcestershire sauce there, because that product contains a trace of anchovy among its ingredients.

There also are no establishments in downtown Loma Linda that sell or serve tobacco and liquor products. When I was growing up, there was not so much as an ashtray to be found anywhere in Loma Linda, not even at the entrances to public buildings. "No Smoking" signs were vigilantly posted everywhere. There never was the slightest whiff of tobacco smoke.

Nor a whiff of beer or whiskey.

Yes, there was a liquor store on Waterman Avenue up by Interstate 10. There was even a dive bar there, called Wayne's Hideaway. Technically, that intersection is in San Bernardino, but it was too close for comfort to Loma Linda. Many a silent prayer was sent up by pious Adventists as they ran the gauntlet there on their way to the freeway.

You should know that I was a red-blooded teenager, so I would slip over to San Bernardino now and then to get my kicks on Route 66. So, I knew what smoke and liquor and meat smelled like. That's why I knew that Loma Linda was different. And special.

Loma Linda runs on a different clock. It not only smells different, but it also looks different and acts different. It's a quiet town. A clean town. A polite town.

I think I became the historic first person ever to utter a swear word there. One day, not long after I had obtained my first driver's license, I got into a dispute with an adult lady over a parking space in front of the Loma Linda Post Office. I was only sixteen and I hadn't yet developed all facets of my now incredible charm. Her rebukes escalated, as did my sarcastic responses, and I ended up telling her to go to hell. She staggered back a step. Then she told ME to go to hell! She staggered back

TWO MORE STEPS! As shocked as she was that I had said it, she was doubly horrified that SHE had said it.

That's Loma Linda for you. Healthy in body, mind, and spirit.

As an insider, though, I now will tell you a dirty little secret about Adventist health.

As good as it is, the Adventist diet could be a lot better, and I'll explain how and why.

It's not much of a secret, really. It pokes out at you everywhere you look in Loma Linda, as well as in other Adventist church bastions around the nation such as Silver Spring, Maryland; Berrien Springs, Michigan; Walla Walla, Washington; and St. Helena, California.

It's flagrant, really. Almost scandalously obvious. It's a situation that can be summed up in two words:

Obese Adventists.

My father, in the days when he was a top church executive, would joke privately about his many fat colleagues. They had "G. C. fronts," he would say, "fronts" meaning bellies and "G. C." meaning General Conference, which is the name of the church's governing body.

Ha! Did I just say "body"? That's a good one!

My father always was stick thin, and so was my mother, but it definitely was a lucky blessing for them, because they both came from families with loads of fat people. Even their own children, including me, have had to fight weight issues most of our lives. We all were born thin, and we grew up thin, but as adults we all got fat. When we were at our heaviest, my siblings and I would look at ourselves, then look at our toothpick parents and joke, "We must be adopted."

Why are many Adventists fat? Here's the explanation:

Although they generally are abstemious or at least moderate in their use of flesh foods and alcohol, they generally are not so abstemious, nor are they moderate, in their use of some other foods. Starchy foods, for example. They love their carbs. And they double up on their carbohydrates with lots of extra sugar. Oh, yes, they love their sugar.

And they love their oils. Oils are just fine, too.

And salt. Lots of salt.

I remember standing in the aisle of the Loma Linda Market one day, checking the labels on cans of various meat substitute products made from soy, gluten, or other plant proteins. Vegeburger, FriChik, Linketts, Nuti-Loaf, Choplets, Skallops . . . the list is long.

The manager at the time was a friend of mine. We graduated in the same class at Loma Linda Academy. He came over to say hello. We shook hands and chatted a bit. Then I started reading him some of the outrageously high salt-content numbers on the cans I had been inspecting. I then asked him, "You call this a health food store?"

I was grinning as I said it. But he didn't grin back. He grimaced.

He knew he was busted!

Mind you, there are plenty of Adventists who do not overdo it on the salt. Or the oils. Or the sugars and starches.

There are plenty of slim Adventists. Millions of them, even.

But there also are millions of Adventists who think nothing of eating potatoes, pasta, rice, and bread—at the same meal. That's a lot of white food, folks. It's very heavy on the carbohydrates, and it weighs very heavy on the people who eat it. Plus, they fry those potatoes in lots of corn oil, and maybe crack a few eggs in there, too, and sprinkle them liberally with salt, and they'll smother the pasta with cheese sauce, and more salt, and sweeten the rice with sugar, and slather the bread with butter. And wash everything down with whole milk. And then there's ice cream for dessert, with plenty of chocolate sauce, caramel syrup, pineapple topping, and sugared coconut flakes on top. Don't forget the candied cherries!

Now, you may have noticed a few items of particular interest in this technically vegetarian menu. I am talking about the eggs, the milk, the butter, the cream, and the cheese. These are animal products.

The vegetarianism of choice for most Adventists, including my own parents and almost all of my extended family, is the form known as lacto-ovo vegetarianism. It means you don't eat the flesh of dead animals, but you're OK with the stuff that comes out of living ones.

It's a sore subject within the church. Vegan Adventists, who shun meat and dairy products both, are an increasingly vocal minority that regularly challenges the lacto-ovo majority to enter into debate on the subject.

It's an argument that goes back to the origins of the church, because the founding prophet Ellen G. White, my great-great-grandmother, seemed to be of two minds on the subject. And she really did deliver a mixed message on this one point.

In her earliest writings on diet, health, and nutrition, she enthusiastically encouraged the use of dairy products, even as she condemned the use of flesh foods.

In later writings, she appeared to be on the verge, at least, of changing her mind.

"The time will come," she wrote in *Counsels on Diet and Foods*, published posthumously in 1938, "when we may have to discard some of the articles of diet we now use, such as milk and cream and eggs."

The bottom line (and a lot of Adventists do have big bottoms as well as big bellies) is that these elite Blue Zoners in Loma Linda and elsewhere could eat better than they do.

That's right, I said it. And I'll say it again, in a different way.

These milk-gulping, cheese-nibbling, egg-swallowing, carbo-loading, salt-shaking, candy-sucking, oil-guzzling lacto-ovo vegetarians live longer and healthier lives than almost everyone else, but just imagine how much longer and healthier their lives might be if they made a few substantial improvements in their diets.

More to the present point, imagine how well *you* could do if you got a head start on them and started outdoing them right now.

Are you imagining it? Is an action plan forming in your head?

Excellent!

This is the positively incredible (and incredibly positive) takeaway message here. As I will demonstrate, you have the power to create a Blue Zone of your own, no matter where you live, and you can turn it as many deeper shades of blue as you like.

In fact, you can have more than a Blue Zone. You can have your own Blue Heaven on Earth!

A Happy Home Remedy That Will Help You Cut Down on Salt

A little salt is good, but too much salt is very, very bad. It causes water retention, raises blood pressure, compromises skin and bone health, and impairs brain, kidney, heart, and stomach function. Between a half teaspoon and a level teaspoon of salt each day is generally considered healthful, depending on a person's age, weight, and overall health. Most people eat far too much. They get hideous amounts of salt in restaurant food. Packaged foods from the market are extremely oversalted, too. Home cooking can be just as bad because, at most people's houses, too much salt goes into the pot, then everyone at the table uses a salt shaker to oversalt the food some more.

According to study results reported in the July 2011 *Proceedings of the National Academy of Sciences*, researchers at Duke University and the University of Melbourne found that salt triggers the release of dopamine, the chemical messenger from the brain's pleasure center to the body. This means that salt actually is addictive in much the same way as alcohol, tobacco, and hard drugs.

Cutting down on salt isn't easy, but you should do it, starting now.

Try flavoring your food with lemon juice, vinegar, or spices. Also, explore the many salt-free seasoning mixes available at stores or online. Or make your own. Here's a simple recipe that's a favorite in my family. We call it Zalt.

ZALT

About ½ cup

3 tablespoons onion powder (not onion salt)
3 tablespoons garlic powder (not garlic salt)
2 tablespoons smoked paprika
1 tablespoon black pepper
1 tablespoon chile powder (optional, for extra kick)

Combine all the ingredients, pour into a shaker or other container, and store in a cool, dry place. Use liberally!

CHAPTER TWO

Health Nut

TO MISQUOTE SHAKESPEARE: SOME ARE BORN TO BE GREAT HEALTH NUTS, some achieve greatness as health nuts, others have greatness as health nuts thrust upon them.

In my case, it's all three.

I am a career journalist who often writes on health, fitness, and nutrition. I have received many honors and commendations for my work in this field, including a national award from the Arthritis Foundation for a lengthy article I did on an innovative camp for arthritic children in the San Bernardino Mountains of Southern California, not far from where I live.

Not only do I write about health, fitness, and nutrition, but I also study these subjects. I keep up with the current research and literature. Many of the facts, figures, and findings cited in this book are culled from other trailblazing books, documentaries, and productions in other media that I admire and recommend, and which I acknowledge in a brief bibliography that is featured among the important closing pages of *The Healthiest People on Earth*.

I can't help but be interested in health topics. It's in my genes. It's in my family, which is loaded from top to bottom with noteworthy health crusaders, including one of the most noteworthy of all time.

My own generation of this family consists of myself and three siblings, plus eight first cousins. That's a fairly small number of people, only a dozen, but it's a group that includes four doctors, two health food store managers, and two executives of a publishing company specializing in health and fitness books. Then there's me, the author of this book. That's nine of twelve, a pretty high percentage of concentrated vocational interest.

We get it from our parents. They, in turn, got it from their parents, who got it from their parents, and so on, going back four generations and more than 150 years to the founding of the Seventh-day Adventist church, a denomination that from the beginning has centered its global ministry on health of body, mind, and spirit.

My father, Howard Benjamin Weeks, was an Adventist minister and singing evangelist who made appearances throughout the country. He even performed at New York City's Carnegie Hall. While still a young man, he was promoted to church administration, becoming the denomination's worldwide director of public relations. This took him to every corner of the globe to promote the church's efforts. He also wrote two books on church ministry and outreach, *Breakthrough* (1962) and *Adventist Evangelism in the 20th Century* (1969). Later he became vice president for public relations and development at the now-famous Loma Linda University School of Medicine and LLU Medical Center, the church's flagship medical school and teaching hospital.

When he retired, he founded his own publishing company, Woodbridge Press, which specialized in books on healthy living. The company catalog included many cookbooks as well as titles on gardening, fitness, and mental health.

My mother, Dorothy White Weeks, had an accomplished career as a nurse and nurse administrator. She wasn't a public figure or an entrepreneur like my father was. On the other hand, she was a member of Adventist royalty, the great-granddaughter of the church's founder and prophet: Ellen G. White. It was because of her that people made such a fuss whenever my family stopped by after church for Sabbath dinner.

My mother and her health-crusading sister, Kathryn White Matheson, the founder in 1959 of one of Southern California's first and best health food stores, Full O' Life Natural Foods in Burbank, were the only children of Herbert Clarence White, Ellen G. White's grandson.

Herbert and his twin brother Henry were longtime missionaries and evangelists, advancing the Adventist message in China and other parts of the world. Herbert also became an author and a publisher. In collaboration with fellow health crusader Dr. H. E. Kirschner, my grandfather wrote such groundbreaking books as *Are You What You Eat?*, *Nature's Seven Doctors*, and *Nature's Healing Grasses*, published under his own imprint, H. C. White Publications, in La Sierra, another Adventist stronghold in Southern California.

My grandfather and his brother were the sons of William Clarence White, known in the family as Willie, who was a lifelong Adventist evangelist and administrator, working tirelessly to promote the church's advocacy of better living through better health.

And why would he not? He was the son of Ellen Gould Harmon White, founder and prophet of the Seventh-day Adventist church and creator of a worldwide movement devoted to the importance of physical and spiritual health. Like all of history's great reformers, she had much to say. She published forty books during her lifetime, and sixty more were collected from her voluminous writings and published after her death in 1915 at the age of eighty-seven.

From almost the beginning of her ministry (it was in 1863 that she and her husband, my great-great-grandfather James White, and their supporters founded the Seventh-day Adventist church), she preached that a sound body is the best foundation for a strong faith. "There are but few as yet who are aroused sufficiently to understand how much their habits of diet have to do with their health, their characters, their usefulness in this world, and their eternal destiny," she wrote in *Testimonies for the Church*, published in 1885.

It's a message that can be found to some extent in virtually all of her books, and it is the core topic of many of them, including *Healthful Living* (1897), *The Ministry of Healing* (1905), *Counsels on Health* (1923), and *Counsels on Diet and Foods* (1938).

In addition to her books, she wrote more than 5,000 articles, all of them in support of the "whole-person" ministry she espoused. She also corresponded ceaselessly with people of all kinds, both inside and outside of the church membership, producing copious numbers of letters that also would end up in print, compiled and published posthumously.

All told, her literary output comes to more than 100,000 pages of text.

Wow.

So, there you have it, the outline of my lineage. It starts at the top with one of history's great health reformers, and works its way down through four generations of other reformers. All the way to me.

Don't worry. I won't be trying to start a new religion on you. One of those rare individuals in a family is quite enough.

Unlike my great-great-grandmother, I don't have a prophetic gift. I don't experience visions. Shoot, even my dreams don't make sense, though they are very entertaining, I must say.

I'm not even cut out to be a preacher. I'm too much of a wise guy for that.

But I certainly am an involved, active, fifth-generation member of a family of notable health crusaders, so I feel it is fair to say this, at least: I am a certifiable health nut.

I not only say it, I claim it as a birthright!

I'm very proud of my ancestry, and humbly indebted to it. It forms me.

Ellen G. White, the grand matriarch of my family, is responsible in so many ways for the way in which I was brought up, and for the manner in which I live. She even is responsible for where I live.

In 1905, she directed that the church invest in property in Loma Linda, originally called Mound City, a small resort town dense with citrus groves located in sunny Southern California. She had received instructions from the Lord, she said, that there was a great destiny and opportunity for the church there.

Later she would recount, "While attending the [church's] General Conference of 1905, at Washington, D.C., I received a letter from

Elder J. A. Burden, describing a property he had found four miles west of Redlands, five and one-half miles southeast of San Bernardino, and eight miles northeast of Riverside. As I read his letter, I was impressed that this was one of the places I had seen in vision, and I immediately telegraphed him to secure the property without delay. He did so, and as the result, Loma Linda is in our possession" (*Loma Linda Messages*, published posthumously in 1935).

Her vision proved to be right on the mark. Loma Linda has become a stronghold of the Adventist church and its global health outreach. Not to mention a Blue Zone.

My father, Howard B. Weeks, brought his family to Loma Linda in 1963 and began his new job as head of development and public relations at Loma Linda University, replacing Jerry L. Pettis, who resigned to seek a seat in the U.S. Congress. My father would become a key architect of the institution's phenomenal growth during the next decade. In 1967, the medical center moved to its present-day quarters in a colossal multi-towered building a few blocks southwest of the original Loma Linda Sanitarium. In August 1971, on a temporary stage constructed outside the still-new medical center, my father and other LLU leaders gathered with Congressman Pettis and California governor Ronald Reagan to welcome President Richard Nixon, who flew in to make the announcement that Loma Linda had been chosen as the site for a new Veterans Administration hospital, replacing the one that had been destroyed earlier that year in the San Fernando Earthquake centered north of Los Angeles.

Not long after this career highlight, my father retired and moved with my mother and my two sisters, Carolyn and Donna, to Santa Barbara, where the new family business, Woodbridge Press, was established. My brother Doug, who graduated with his medical degree from LLU and joined the faculty there, eventually accepted career opportunities that took him elsewhere, and he left Loma Linda, too.

I am the only one in our family who remains here. I have lived in or near Loma Linda for fifty years now.

I'm still in the zone.

The Blue Zone.

And, remember, you can be in the zone, too.

No, you don't have to move to Loma Linda and live with me (though feel free to send a photo and perhaps we'll talk).

As I said before, I'm going to tell you, and show you, how to create a space for yourself, a zone of your own, wherever you happen to be, that will help you reach your highest potential for a healthy life, a long life, and a good life.

A Happy Home Remedy for Whatever Ails You (According to My Grandfather)

I grew up knowing all about the famous "Green Drink," a concoction that was promoted as an all-purpose health tonic, capable of boosting energy, cleansing the blood, aiding digestion, and correcting "diseases of malnutrition and physical degeneration." That's a quote from the book *Nature's Healing Grasses* (1960), a collaboration between H. E. Kirschner and my grandfather Herbert C. White. There's a whole chapter titled "The Therapeutic 'Green Drink,'" that tells how Dr. Kirschner developed the beverage as a restorative for tuberculosis patients he was treating in the 1930s at Olive View Sanitorium in Sylmar, near Los Angeles (which grew to become today's Olive View UCLA Medical Center).

Kirschner and my grandfather were great believers in the "Green Drink" not only as a cure but also as a preventive to be taken every day.

Here's the recipe for a single serving:

DR. KIRSCHNER'S THERAPEUTIC GREEN DRINK

Serves 1

2 cups unsweetened pineapple juice, divided

15 almonds, soaked overnight in water

5 teaspoons sunflower seeds, soaked overnight in water

4 pitted dates, soaked overnight in water

4 large handfuls assorted greens such as parsley, mint, spinach, beet greens, watercress, kale, chard, alfalfa, and dandelion

1. In a blender, combine 1 cup of the unsweetened pineapple juice with the softened nuts, seeds, and dates. Blend well.
2. Add the remaining 1 cup unsweetened pineapple juice plus the greens and blend again until all is liquefied.
3. Drink immediately or refrigerate to chill.

CHAPTER THREE

As I Lay Dieting

I WAS SHOCKED THE FIRST TIME I SAW A PHOTO OF MYSELF THAT SHOWED ME looking fat.

I was twenty years old. I was viewing the slides that my bride and I had taken on our honeymoon. One of her shots showed me emerging from the ocean, sputtering, hair hanging in my face, with what looked like a tubby stomach hanging over the elastic of my Hawaiian-print swim jams.

"I look like a whale!" I complained. "Let's get rid of that one."

"Why?" my ridiculously skinny bride asked.

"It's a bad angle. Or bad lighting or something. I don't look like that," I explained.

My bride patted my hand reassuringly. She said, "Yes, you do."

Wow. I had heard that it's common for people to gain weight after they get married. But I figured it took longer than a few days!

Oh, well. A honeymoon is as good a time as any, I suppose, to discover that life is full of nasty surprises. And, honestly, it was pretty easy, at first, to turn the tables on this particular nasty surprise. I found that I could lose belly fat almost as quickly, if not more quickly, than I gained it.

I did it by resorting occasionally to that righteous biblical practice known as fasting.

It's amazing to think back on it, because now I can't last a single food-free day without feeling that death is drawing near, but in my twenties it was easy. As long as there was plenty of good cold Arrowhead Springs drinking water to be had, I could go three, four, five, even six days without a morsel of solid food.

I usually would break my fast on Friday evening, when dinner with my wife's family was a weekly tradition. I offhandedly would announce that I had lost ten pounds since we had gathered at the table a week earlier.

My mother-in-law, a wonderful Adventist woman whose skills as a cook always interfered with her efforts as a dieter, would respond with some affectionate remark along the lines of, "You make me sick!"

Over time, though, my fasting superpowers waned. And, sadly, the propensity of my body to gain weight did not wane in the least. Indeed, it waxed forth prodigiously.

My eating habits were changing, because my lifestyle in general was changing. I was out of my family home now and establishing a home of my own. I had an Adventist wife, and she did her heroic best, God knows, to keep me in line, but I had a questing spirit and a curious mind. I wanted to put my newfound independence to use and explore the world's possibilities. And sample its pleasures.

I transferred from the Adventist college where I had spent my freshman year to the decidedly secular University of California at Riverside. I gained employment in the secular world of journalism, landing a full-time job in the newsroom of the daily *San Bernardino Sun*. My circle of friends became more secular. I formed new bonds with a whole new demographic: non-Adventists.

We all are influenced by our surroundings, so it's no surprise that I started thinking and talking and acting and eating a little more like the people in this new secular world around me, and a little less like the people in the parochial world in which I had grown up.

My Adventist root system took another hit when, in our thirties, my long-suffering Adventist wife gave up on me, and we divorced. A few years later, I married an excellent non-Adventist woman who was a journalist like myself and who worked where I worked.

Our combined income was a good one, and we could afford a few nice things. We became quite the sophisticates, with a proper appreciation of epicurean food and fine wine. We started shopping at those high-end "foodie" markets. We arranged our travel schedule around various "fancy food" shows. We were regulars at all the local food and wine galas. We subscribed to several monthly mail-order wine clubs.

We were sitting pretty.

And pretty heavy, at that.

We had a large circle of like-minded friends who became our co-conspirators in many feasting and imbibing adventures. We even started what we called a gourmet club, destined to last for years, in which we and several other couples took turns hosting a monthly themed dinner at our various homes. The rule was that the host couple would prepare the main dish, and each of the other couples would prepare and bring a single, theme-appropriate side dish.

This rule routinely was broken. The host couple usually put on a whole spread, while each guest couple would bring two or three sides, so these monthly gastronomic rampages were epic in scale. During an occasion when my wife and I hosted a dinner with a Native American theme, one of my personal culinary triumphs was grilled elk steaks with a juniper berry reduction sauce, served with great quantities of a red wine of which I have no memory whatsoever, except that it was stupendously expensive.

As I evolved from my thirties into my forties, I found that my figure was evolving, too. Fasting was no longer an option. A young body can go for days without food, but an older body?

Not so much.

I found myself forced to explore other forms of dieting.

I remember one that was quite popular—the Beverly Hills Diet. It was a favorite among the female members of my extended family. It was pretty much an all-fruit diet, and I gave it a try now and then. Hey,

I love fruit, and it's fun to cut up big bowlfuls of mango, pineapple, strawberries, plums, melons, and cherries. If I remember correctly, you could eat any kind of fruit you liked, and as much of it as you liked. It was an awesome diet. For a while.

But then, as always happens, the too-much-of-a-good-thing factor kicks in. And let's face it, if you're eating that much fruit, you probably are eating way too much sugar, even if it is natural sugar. And, for sure, with all that squishy fruit flesh in your system, and not much else, you are excusing yourself a little too often to go to the bathroom.

Then, there was the grapefruit and egg diet. It brought something new to the table that hadn't been part of the all-fruit diet. Namely, something that wasn't fruit. And yet, there were fewer choices. You could have your grapefruit with boiled eggs or scrambled eggs or fried eggs or poached eggs. That's about the whole list of possibilities right there, as I recall.

I tried every diet there is. In fact, just this second I Googled "fad diets" and a listing popped up of the "Worst Diets of All Time." Sure enough, I checked each one and nodded ruefully. Been there, done that. I've tried almost every single one of them.

The one that made me feel the worst is one that has been in and out of fashion for many years. Many people swear by it. Others swear at it. It calls for drinking a witch's brew of water, maple syrup, cayenne pepper, and lemon as your only source of nourishment for as many days or weeks as you can bear.

I was only into the second day of it when I started to feel weak, sick, and nauseated. On the third day, I called my brother Doug, the doctor, and told him what I was doing.

He told me, with the kind of forcefulness that suggested he physically was trying to reach through my phone receiver and shake me by the neck, that this diet was woefully lacking in nutrition. I must STOP IT IMMEDIATELY.

I stopped it immediately.

Hey, brother doctor's orders!

Oh, I tried many other diets, too. I experimented with different versions of the all-protein diet. And I tried a few all-carbohydrate diets. There was one called the bread diet, and you could eat anything you wanted to eat, as long as it was in a sandwich. The idea was to eat lots and lots of bread. I think I gained fifteen pounds in a week on that one.

Let's see, what else did I try? I always have been an adventurous sort. I always have been willing to give anything a shot.

Of course I tried the one-big-meal-a-day diet. And the six-small-meals-a-day diet. I tried every sort of calorie-counting system and portion-control plan. I chewed what were billed as appetite-suppressing caramels, and I thought they were delicious, especially when they were combined with a mammoth meal. I ate meal-replacement nutrition bars that were so gooey and sweet that I'm sure they contained two or three meals' worth of bad stuff.

I purchased a membership in an internet diet club, with a secret password and everything, where I could access total meal plans for every day of the week, every week of the month, every month of the year, forever and ever.

I was impressed by the menus. They were good. And I am confident that, over time, they would have offered tangible benefits. Trouble is, they were so complicated, and they involved so much grocery buying, in small increments, that I soon concluded that buying and preparing and eating food would take over my whole schedule. And my whole paycheck.

I hear similar complaints about many of the most famous weight-loss programs. They cost too much. They take up too much time. They are too complicated. They require too much work.

Frankly, it's stupid to waste time and money this way. Eating is not the purpose of life. It's quite the other way around. Life is the purpose of eating.

That's right, we eat in order to live. We do not live in order to eat.

A lot of people are confused about this. They have it ass-backward, and you can tell by looking at their asses.

Believe me, I am saying this with a heart full of love and compassion, because I have been among the lost and confused. In fact, I don't think I became "unconfused," if that's a word, until the year my parents died of natural causes, three months apart, each at the dignified age of eighty-nine.

I delivered the eulogy at both of their funerals. And, thinking about what to say, and in writing down my thoughts, I reflected in a clear, linear way about their lives, and their lineage, and about my connection to them, and to that lineage.

And then, later, I viewed the pictures taken at those funerals, which included shots of this fat guy—and by "fat guy" I mean me—paying tribute to my skinny parents, and charting their places of honor in a proud line of notable health crusaders.

And I asked myself one question.

What in the hell is wrong with me?

Why have I been beating around bushes for years trying to find answers that have been right in front of me all along?

I mean, in back of me.

Yes, I needed to get back, get back, get back to where I once belonged. (Uh-oh, do I owe Paul McCartney some money now?)

I realized that my best way forward was to circle around and return to my roots. I needed to rediscover that the best way to eat is the way I was brought up to eat.

And, in making this rediscovery, I also discovered something else. Something new and wonderful.

I discovered that the diet of my youth, as good as it was, could be significantly improved. I could eat even better than I did as a kid. I could eat even better than my parents did. Dare I say it? I could eat even better than my great-great-grandmother did!

Yes, I discovered that I could eat what is the most nutritious, most delicious, most inexpensive, most uncomplicated, most time-saving, easiest-to-prepare diet that is available on our planet.

We will call it the World's Best Diet.

A Happy Home Remedy for Snack Attacks

My parents never went on diets. In fact, they were grazers who ate all day, every day. They ate three full meals, plus they nibbled on snacks between meals. And they were slender their entire lives. How is this possible? Well, they ate sensible portions at meal-time, and then, when they got the munchies between meals, they snacked on good things, not bad things. I never, ever saw them scarfing chips out of a bag, or sneaking cookies and candy, or scooping up a dish of mid-afternoon ice cream, or heating up pizza rolls or puff pastries. No, they nibbled on fresh veggies, fruits, and nuts.

They always kept cucumbers and bunches of carrots and celery in the fridge, and they would cut these up to make nutritious snack sticks. No dip, except maybe a little peanut butter if they were feeling wild and wicked.

A whole long countertop in their kitchen usually was loaded with fruit. No kidding, it looked like a farmers' market in there. Bananas next to papayas next to oranges next to apples next to grapes and more. And there always was a nut dish or two around the house. Every kind of nut. Even Brazil nuts. My dad loved those.

I often think of my dad and mom when I reach for a snack. They were smart. They knew how to do it. Snacking on fresh, nutritious foods offers a double advantage. It's good for you. So, you can do more of it!

CHAPTER FOUR

The World's Best Diet

I AM NOT GOING TO USE THE WORD "VEGAN" IN THIS CHAPTER.

Well, except for just now, I guess. But that's it.

My friend Tamara Thorne, the horror novelist, who is very good at scaring people, especially me, has warned me that I'll lose a lot of readers if I use the word "vegan."

Oops. I said it again.

I respect Tamara's advice, and I fear her wrath if I ignore it, so rest assured, you won't be hearing the word "vegan" out of me!

Oops.

Apparently, I need to resort to alternative wording so that I won't keep making this mistake.

How about "plant-based"? Does that work?

OK, let me use it in a sentence: A plant-based whole foods diet has the power to improve health, protect against disease, and prolong life.

There you have it, the single most important sentence in this book, in all its alternatively worded glory.

What does "plant-based" mean? It refers to any food that springs forth from planet Earth, whether in trees or on bushes or among vines or upon the soil, whether in gardens, fields, orchards, or wild thickets. It refers to every food there is, in fact, except for the flesh or bodily discharges of our companion creatures, the animals and birds and insects and fish with whom we share the planet.

What does the term "whole foods" mean? It refers to foods that are intact in their original state and are not processed or modified or altered in ways that compromise their natural nutritional goodness. Sometimes it takes vigilance to locate and identify whole foods. A loaf of bread labeled "whole wheat" may sound healthier than bleached white bread, and it is, but most so-called "whole wheat" breads are made from refined wheat flour, which makes the word "whole" misleading. Look for bread that is labeled "whole grain whole wheat." That's the far better choice.

Checking labels is a good thing. Vigilance is worthwhile, because eating a plant-based whole foods diet will strengthen your body and maximize your health.

It's proven truth. The studies have been done. The evidence is in.

A prominent example of the research in this field is the China-Oxford-Cornell Diet and Health Project conducted over the course of three decades and published in book form in 2006 as *The China Study*. Considered the most scientifically rigorous investigation ever undertaken of the relationship between nutrition and health (the *New York Times* called it the "Grand Prix of epidemiology"), the China Study compared the meat-based diet favored in America and other Western nations with the plant-based diet that predominates in much of the Asian world. It found that, simply put, a meat diet results in poor health and a plant diet results in good health.

Says the study's director, Dr. T. Colin Campbell of Cornell University, "The consumption of whole, plant-based foods offers the best strategy for creating health and preventing serious diseases."

Another long-term study, led by one of America's most distinguished surgeons, the Cleveland Clinic's Dr. Caldwell B. Esselstyn Jr., resulted in the 1995 book *Prevent and Reverse Heart Disease*. His research found that heart disease patients actually can be saved by purely nutritional intervention.

Says Dr. Esselstyn, "We recruited patients who had basically been told to go home and prepare for death, and put them on a plant-based diet. Every one of them who followed the diet lived without any more incidence of heart disease."

In fact, the results of his work have led Esselstyn to make the boldest of claims: "Cardiovascular disease is an absolutely toothless paper tiger that need never exist, and if it does exist it need never progress. It is a food-borne illness. Change your food, and you change your life."

These are impressive words from an impressive source, a former president of the American Association of Endocrine Surgeons and the inaugural recipient, in 2005, of the Benjamin Spock Award for Compassion in Medicine.

The work of Esselstyn and Campbell is featured in the compelling film documentary *Forks Over Knives* (2011) directed by Lee Fulkerson. The film also showcases the work and testimony of many other well-known health and nutrition experts. And we hear, too, from many survivors of deadly diseases who tell their stories of diet-based recovery.

The narrative builds to one conclusion: Most of the degenerative diseases that plague humanity can be prevented, controlled, even reversed by choosing plant-based nutrition. What we do for ourselves with our forks can do more wonders by far than what surgeons can do for us with their knives.

As I said, the evidence is in. And, interestingly, it backs up the prescient statements about health and nutrition made by my great-great-grandmother, Ellen G. White, more than a hundred years ago. Though her words are framed in the context of her ministry, they convey a powerful health message that stands alone.

"Again and again I have been shown that God is bringing His people back to His original design, that is, not to subsist upon the flesh of dead animals. He would have us teach people a better way," she wrote. "Grains, fruits, nuts, and vegetables constitute the diet chosen for us by our Creator. These foods, prepared in as simple and natural manner as possible, are the most healthful and nourishing. They impart a strength, a powerful endurance, and a vigor of intellect" (*Ministry of Healing*, 1905).

Modern science is proving beyond doubt the truth of these words. The meaty diet most Americans eat today is loaded with fat and cholesterol, poisons that cause obesity and promote the onset and growth of heart disease, cancer, and stroke (America's number 1, 2, and 3 leading causes of death, respectively), as well as other diseases such as diabetes, osteoporosis, multiple sclerosis, and Alzheimer's disease, which also are on the list of America's top killers.

Animal protein thickens our blood and promotes the formation of plaque that clogs the pipes through which the blood flows, creating a double burden on our cardiovascular system. Studies also show that animal protein creates a hostile acidic environment in our bodies in which cancer cells and other disease cells thrive.

Considering the proven link between all these deadly diseases and nutrition, it's fair to state that most meat eaters die poisoned by the food that they eat.

Americans spend more than $2 trillion each year on health care. That's four times the size of the national defense budget. But we don't have better health in return for our investment. In fact, the World Health Organization reports that America's health care system is among the worst performers on Earth. Despite all the dollars, despite all the advances in modern medicine and surgery, we are sicker than ever. The plain fact is that we are wrecking our bodies faster than they can be repaired.

Even when our poor food choices don't kill us, they cause us much suffering. A diet loaded with unhealthy fats and oils, chemical additives, salt, sugar, nutrient-stripped calories, and other junk has been implicated scientifically with such diverse ailments as arthritis, lupus, renal stones, migraines and other headaches, constipation and irritable bowel syndrome, insomnia, chronic fatigue, PMS, asthma, cataracts, erectile dysfunction, infertility, allergies, skin diseases, even acne.

Even dandruff.

Think about it. Everything from killer diseases to pesky nuisances like acne and dandruff are linked directly to the food we eat.

It's a big problem, which is a bad thing, but there's a ready solution, which is a good thing. Food can be the hero in our lives instead of the villain. All we have to do is eat better food and, snap, it's like pulling a switch that shuts down all those deadly diseases and bothersome conditions.

Just like that.

Changing our diet is a change we need to make. And it's a change we must make if we want to live to our full potential as the human inhabitants of planet Earth. (If you are not a member of this important demographic group, please return this book promptly for a full refund!)

What does "changing our diet" mean? Well, it means more than some people think.

For example, there is little comfort to be found in modern research for those who make a distinction between flesh foods and dairy foods. Eggs, for example, are full of fat and cholesterol and all the other stuff that goes into making birds with feathers, gizzards, beaks, and claws. You don't need any of that fowl stuff inside of you. Your own body produces all the fat and cholesterol you can handle safely. If you're adding fat and cholesterol from the bodies of other creatures, you're squawking for trouble.

And milk? Campbell, director of the China Study, grew up on a dairy farm and believed with all his heart in the wholesome goodness of milk. That is, until he grew up and became a great scientist who conducted research that showed that casein, the main protein in milk, is toxic to humans. Campbell found that he actually was able to turn the growth of cancer cells on or off by raising or lowering doses of casein in laboratory studies.

"Let there be no doubt: Cow milk protein is an exceptionally potent cancer promoter," he says. "It's the most significant carcinogen we consume." Take heed, all you milk-glugging, cheese-scarfing lacto-ovo vegetarians!

Including you Seventh-day Adventist ones!

There also is no comfort in modern research for the rationalizing carnivores who cling to the belief, or maybe it's just a hope, that white meat is better than red meat, or that fish flesh is more healthy to eat than mammal flesh, or that there are special virtues in eating organic meat, grass-fed meat, or free-range meat.

Alas, it's all meat. It's the flesh of dead animal creatures. It all contains destructive animal proteins, cholesterol, and fats that sicken and kill humans, and none of the essential dietary fiber, aminos, and anti-oxidants that strengthen humans and protect them from disease and early death.

No matter what kind of animal creature it is, or how it was raised and fed and perhaps even pampered, it still is a dead animal when we eat it. "The protein is the same," Campbell says.

The trouble is not to be found in the quality of flesh foods, he says, but in the simple fact that it is "that kind of food."

My great-great-grandmother said much the same thing, a long time ago. In the early years of her ministry, when she began preaching the virtues of a vegetarian diet, Ellen G. White did make allowances for fish and fowl. She even partook of these foods herself on occasion. But in time she received inspiration to believe that flesh foods of all kinds are to be avoided. In an 1898 letter to Dr. John Harvey Kellogg, she wrote, "There is no safety in eating of the flesh of dead animals, and in a short time the milk of the cows will too be excluded from the diet of God's commandment-keeping people. It will not be safe to use anything that comes from the animal creation."

Today, it's not just that we eat bad food that is the problem. It's that we eat so much more of it than we used to.

The figures show that a century ago, Americans ate about 120 pounds of meat per person each year. Today, we eat about 200 pounds of meat each year, almost twice as much.

We used to eat less than 300 pounds of dairy products each year. Now, it's more than 600 pounds, more than twice as much.

Animal products aren't the only culprits. Americans once consumed about 40 pounds of processed sugar per person each year. Today, it's almost 150 pounds, almost four times as much.

When the federal Centers for Disease Control and Prevention con-ducted its first national health survey, in the early 1960s, it determined that about one-fourth of all Americans were overweight as measured against a standard body-mass index. At that time, the fledgling fast-food revolution was just a little more than a decade old, having begun in 1948 with the first McDonald's drive-in in San Bernardino, California.

Of course, the fast-food industry has burgeoned since then, and so has the size of Americans. On average we weigh in excess of 20 pounds more than we did in the 1960s. Fat people are now a full three-quarters majority. (That's right, I said full.) The percentage of overweight adults has more than doubled. So has the percentage of overweight children ages six to eleven. The percentage of overweight adolescents ages twelve to nineteen has more than tripled. Obesity is an epidemic that is fueling epidemic-scale rates of diabetes and other degenerative diseases.

We keep getting bigger, and our food keeps getting junkier. New innovations in nutrient-robbing food processing have added to the problem. So has the development of sweeteners and other additives like high fructose corn syrup that were unknown in previous decades.

So has the advent of "super-sized" food merchandising and promotion. In the early years of fast food, a typical bag of french fries contained 200 calories. Now, it's 500. Sodas used to be 8 ounces, with about 75 calories. Now, we can gulp soft drinks that are four times that size or even bigger. A hamburger used to be a single patty on a single bun. A cheeseburger had a single slice of cheese. Now, we see hamburgers that consist of four beef patties and four slices of cheese, plus bacon and eggs and sometimes lots of other things, all of it loaded into a tower that also includes multiple layers of nutritionally dead bread and globs of sweet, fatty sauce.

I usually go to the Los Angeles County Fair each year, and I usually enjoy some of the culinary indulgences commonly found at local and state fairs. But what a difference a few years makes! I remember when popcorn, cotton candy, and an icy snow cone were the available temptations. Today, those treats certainly still exist, but there also are new culinary monstrosities such as deep-fried candy bars, deep-fried snack cakes, and deep-fried ice cream sandwiches. On a stick.

Newly introduced at the last L.A. County Fair I attended was a deep-fried doughnut Sloppy Joe. That's a hamburger patty and cheese enclosed not in a bun but in a glazed doughnut, then topped with beef chili, then plunged into deep-fry oil to create a molten mass of astronomical gastronomical peril.

I checked online to see what's going on at other fairs around the nation, and I learned there are other concoctions that are just as scary. The Oklahoma State Fair, for example, offers what it calls the Pancake Burger, which is a half-pound beef patty topped with peanut butter, bacon, a fried egg, and syrup, all squeezed between two pancakes instead of a bun.

You can find Deep-Fried Butter Balls at the Montana State Fair, Chocolate-Coated Corn Dogs With Candy Sprinkles at the Orange County Fair in California, and a Hot Beef Sundae at the Iowa State Fair that consists of buttery mashed potatoes posing as ice cream, beef gravy standing in as chocolate, and heaps of cheddar cheese playing the role of butterscotch sauce.

Oh, dear. Considering the food we are willing and eager to eat, it's small wonder that we are so fat and sick.

Here's the big wonder: Why don't we make the one instant change that stops our crazy carnival ride to an early grave?

We can stop it in a second.

As the research shows, a plant-based whole foods diet of fresh fruits, vegetables, leafy greens, whole grains, nuts, and legumes keeps the body clean and lean, and prevents, moderates, even reverses almost all the diseases and ailments that make our lives miserable, that shorten or even cost us our lives.

So, why don't all of us make the switch right now? What are we waiting for? Is there something wrong with our heads?

Well, yes, in fact there is.

We are brainwashed.

We are creatures of habit. We are comfortable with our deadly diets. And we literally are afraid of the healthy diet.

It's too different, we think. It takes too much extra time and effort, we think. It costs more, and we don't get our money's worth, we think. We don't get enough protein and other nutrients, we think.

You know what?

Baloney!

Plant foods provide all the protein we need, and that protein is better for us than animal protein. Grains, nuts, and legumes are loaded with the stuff. Even plant foods that are not commonly regarded as protein-packed nevertheless deliver sufficient quantities to supply our needs. Take potatoes, for example. A hearty potato baked in its skin has 5 grams of protein. That's more than what is found in one of those long skinny beefstick sausages that you see at the convenience store. Check it out.

It is completely unnecessary to consume the flesh of dead animals or the secretions of living ones in order to keep ourselves protein-strong. Plant foods do it all. And they do a better job of it.

It's just as easy to debunk the other superstitions about a plant-based whole foods diet. Here goes:

- **"IT TAKES TOO MUCH TIME AND EFFORT."** Really? Tell you what. You go fire up the barbecue and grill some hamburgers. I'll make a big hearty salad loaded with good stuff. Let's see who finishes first.
- **"IT'S TOO EXPENSIVE."** Really? Fill up your grocery cart in the produce department and skip the meat aisle for a while, then start counting the savings. You'll be amazed.
- **"IT'S TOO DIFFERENT. IT'S TOO WEIRD."** Really? Vegetarians don't eat bugs, or things out of the ocean that look like bugs. Vegetarians don't eat liver, which is basically the filter in an animal. It's like eating cigarette butts, or the dirty pads from an air-conditioning unit. Vegetarians don't eat frog legs or pig feet or sheep testicles or cow cheeks. Vegetarians don't eat tongue. Ew. Eating tongue is like French-kissing a cow. I mean, who are the real weirdos here?
- **"A PLANT-BASED WHOLE FOODS DIET IS TOO BLAND, TOO BORING."** Really? Check out the meat counter at your market. It's all the same stuff. It's just different pieces of dead animal. The colors are drab. And the place stinks. Now, go to the produce department. It smells good! Look at all the colors! Ravishing

red radishes and apples and beets. Sunshiny yellow lemons and bananas and squashes. Opulent orange tangerines and pumpkins and carrots. Gorgeous green limes and artichokes and honeydews. Royal purple eggplants and grapes. Beautiful blue potatoes and blueberries. So many choices! Luscious fruits and berries, crunchy vegetables, chewy nuts and legumes, fragrant greens. It's like a banquet for the senses!

And, mind you, nature's bounty is available everywhere, and year-round, not only in grocery stores but also at farmers' markets, at community gardens, and through farm-to-table cooperatives that are to be found throughout the world. One example is Community Supported Agriculture (CSA), which has programs in all fifty of the United States and every province of Canada. (More information: www.nal.usda.gov/ afsic/community-supported-agriculture.)

Of course, you also can grow a lot of your own produce, wherever you live, and whatever the season. Ellen G. White was an avid home gardener and she lived for much of her life in the harsh-winter climes of Maine and Michigan!

There's a whole chapter about gardening coming up later in this book, with lots of stories, tips, and other good information. Meanwhile, though, let's bring this chapter to its ringing conclusion.

Plant-based nutrition is abundant and full of blessings, my friends. It is much more than a diet. It's a whole new way of living better, living stronger, living longer.

Should we even call it a diet? It's almost the opposite of a diet! You can stop getting so stressed out over calorie counts. And portion controls. Seriously.

Once you stop loading up on bad food, you'll find that you can load up on all the good food you want. That's right. All you can eat.

What's for breakfast? How about whole-grain buckwheat griddle cakes mounded high with crushed strawberries and toasted almond slivers? Or maybe Scottish oatmeal topped with blueberries, banana slices, and cashews, perhaps drizzled with a little maple syrup?

What's for lunch? Avocado tacos with Mexican slaw and red chile sauce would be nice. So would grilled portobello mushroom burgers with sweet potato fries. Or a chilled bulgur wheat salad with colorful confetti-chopped veggies, savory chickpeas, parsley, and lemon.

What's for dinner? Try spicy black bean enchiladas loaded with grilled corn kernels, red onion, black olives, and chopped cilantro. Or spinach, mushroom, and cashew lasagna. Or a layered eggplant, zucchini, and tomato casserole.

Side dishes? How about garlicky smashed potatoes with chives and toasted pine nuts? Or a beautiful broccoli, pecan, and cranberry salad? The possibilities are limitless. (And yes, if you're wondering, you will find recipes for all of these dishes in the back pages of this book.)

Oh, what's for dessert? How about peach and rhubarb cobbler with caramelized pecans? Or maybe fresh fruit kebabs dipped in rich dark chocolate?

Does all this sound good?

It is good.

And it's easy.

Honest.

Think of it like this. If you always have been a meat-and-potatoes person, congratulations, you only will have to ditch one of those things. See? You're already halfway to being a vegan!

Damn, I said "vegan" again.

A Happy Home Remedy for the Diet-Change Jitters

Nervous about going meat-free? Don't be. Remind yourself as often as needed that there's only one kind of food that's now off the table: animal products. Everything else is OK. Everything. What could be more doable?

- **GOING MEAT-FREE IS DOABLE AT HOME.** You're in charge of the menu and meal preparation, and you have a whole world of wonderful foods from which to choose.

- **GOING MEAT-FREE IS DOABLE AT RESTAURANTS.** Not only are there growing numbers of vegetarian and vegan restaurants, plus ethnic restaurants with signature meat-free dishes, but also more and more conventional restaurants are sensing a trend and adding new vegetarian options to their menus. Even the most stubbornly carnivorous restaurants have a few righteous items, whether they like it or not, including pasta dishes and salads.
- **GOING MEAT-FREE IS DOABLE EVEN AT FAST-FOOD RESTAURANTS.** It's true. Even the drive-thrus, no matter how short and meat-centric their menus may be, can be navigated successfully. I will vouch for it personally. If I'm away from home and in need of a quick breakfast, I love the Fruit and Maple Oatmeal at McDonald's. I ask for it without cream, and with extra fruit and berries. If I'm stuck for lunch somewhere, I'll stop in at Wendy's for a baked potato with onions and salsa. For an on-the-go dinner, a big bean burrito at Del Taco or Taco Bell will do the trick. Both chains claim their beans and tortillas are lard-free. The folks behind the counter usually are happy, if I ask them nicely, to skip the cheese and instead pack my burrito with chopped onions, diced tomatoes, and shredded lettuce. I ask for extra hot sauce, too. *Muy bueno!*

Here's another trick that works at almost any fast food restaurant. Order a hamburger or other meat sandwich . . . without the meat. A nice juicy tomato sandwich with pickles, onions, and lettuce ain't bad!

CHAPTER FIVE

Cheating in Moderation

RELAX. IT'S NOT LIKE YOU CAN'T EVER, EVER EAT A BIG MAC AGAIN.

A little responsible cheating now and then isn't going to kill you, if it's done in moderation.

Note the key words here: "moderation," "now and then," "responsible," "a little."

Of course, you might be one of those people who can't cheat at all without running off the rails and crashing. For those people, a little cheating leads immediately to lots of cheating, and then cheating all the time. That won't work. If you are one of those all-or-nothing people, you better go "all in" on health and choose "nothing" when it comes to temptation, at least until you can trust yourself a bit more.

If you're like most people, though, you actually might benefit from a moderate amount of responsible cheating. It's easier to get through that first week of diet change if you know there's a little sinful indulgence waiting for you on the weekend. Eventually, as you purify your system, you probably will come to regard that indulgence as less and less important, or even appealing. Take it a week at a time. Then, take it a month at a time. It may be easier, for a while, to get through the first twenty-nine or thirty days of the month if there's a naughty prize waiting on the last day. Don't be surprised if that temptation, too, starts to subside over time.

I don't indulge in "scheduled" cheating anymore. I don't need it. On the other hand, I don't beat myself up if I occasionally eat a slice of combination pizza with cheese and all the toppings at a friend's house while watching a football game. It's OK, because the rest of my snacking during the game is of the righteous kind. I will have brought plenty of veggie sticks and hummus, or whole-grain crackers and pesto sauce, or tortilla chips and guacamole, or popcorn and sliced apples and grapes. Good stuff like that.

I don't get down on myself if I occasionally eat a hamburger, if I'm traveling by car and I get hungry in a town where the only chow is McDonald's. It's OK, because 999 times out of a thousand, I get hungry in towns where there are plenty of other choices. And, by the way, I am noticing with satisfaction that even some of the fast-food chains are starting to offer veggie burgers and other similar options. It's about time!

I don't hang my head if I occasionally have a hot date night at a fancy restaurant and decide to go nuts. Hey, just because I'm a health nut doesn't mean I can't be a nut in other ways now and then! Not long ago I visited a Southern California restaurant famous for its seafood. It also offers vegetarian fare, which is what I usually order, but this time my companion chose a seafood dish, and I did, too. I ordered the snowy white scallops, and they arrived perfectly cooked and served with aromatic rice and steamed vegetables. The meal was quite lovely.

And it was guilt-free, too, as far as I was concerned, because it had been months since I had eaten seafood, and it will be many more months before I eat it again.

That's the key, you see. Cheat in moderation. It can serve as a safety feature, a handy-if-needed pressure valve. You don't have to chafe against a rigid "never again" policy. If you say yes to temptation on rare occasions, it makes it easy to say no thanks on all the other occasions.

Also, a short detour to the wild side carries its own corrective reminder, I have found. A little meat always messes up my digestion and leaves me feeling a little worse for wear. It's a helpful admonition that underlines the fact that a plant-based whole foods diet is the way to go, day in and day out.

It's like the wooziness you feel after a gut-wrenching thrill ride at the amusement park. It might have been a blast while it was happening, but you figure it's going to be a while before you want to do it again!

I never will forget the time I ate my first morsel of meat. It definitely was a cheating situation.

I was about ten years old, which means my younger brother Doug, who also has a role in this story, was about seven. One day, during a vacation stay at the home of loved ones, our Uncle Floyd took all of us kids bowling, which was exciting enough, but then, after we all were good and tired and hungry, he bought us hamburgers at the lunch counter. That's right—real beef hamburgers.

Uncle Floyd, the husband of my father's sister Jean, was a wonderful man, and we kids adored him. He always had a little mischief in him, even though he was a solid, upstanding Adventist. He told us funny stories, and teased us, and made faces at us. There always was a twinkle in his eye. He let us stay up late on Saturday nights to watch wrestling on TV. One night he even surprised us with a six-pack of Near Beer. We all felt very adult and sophisticated as we sipped our Near Beer and watched Gorgeous George throwing his opponents around.

Of course, there is no appreciable alcohol in Near Beer. But there definitely is meat in a hamburger, so buying hamburgers at the bowling alley was Uncle Floyd's craziest stunt ever! Naturally, my brother and I were thrilled. Our cousins, it turned out, were old pros when it came to eating the occasional hamburger. They were nonchalant and cool about it. But for Doug and me, this was a breathtaking rite of passage. We ate our burgers very solemnly, nodding with approval like true gourmets, and we pretended to think they were supremely delicious, even though they weren't at all.

Later, when we returned to the house, Doug couldn't wait a second before he announced to the other members of our assembled families, "We ate REAL HAM hamburgers!"

He may or may not have known the difference between beef and ham, as innocent as he was, but he was making the declaration for effect, anyway. The word "hamburger" has the word "ham" in it, and "ham" was a bad word in my family.

Was my Uncle Floyd mortified at being busted like this? Oh, heck no. He laughed his head off. In fact, he would retell the story of the "REAL HAM hamburgers" a thousand times during the rest of his long life, and howl with laughter each time. He lived to be ninety years old.

My dad thought it was funny, too.

Mom? She was horrified, of course.

Mom and Dad were different that way. Dad had grown up in the sticks of rural Arizona and Texas in a dirt-poor Adventist family that sometimes had to shoot or catch the food they ate. He would continue to eat a little meat, now and then, for most of his life, though never at home and rarely in my mother's presence.

Mom, on the other hand, had grown up in the Adventist royal family, as it were, and she never knowingly ate so much as one morsel of meat in her entire life. (We kept our silence on those occasions when she would puzzle over the mystery ingredients in whatever so-called vegetarian dishes we were served at this or that ethnic restaurant.)

Mom and Dad were only days apart in age, and they both lived to the age of eighty-nine, dying within three months of each other, so it wouldn't seem that my dad lost any advantage due to the little bit of meat that he ate, or that my mom gained any advantage for never touching the stuff. It worked out to be a tie.

Remember, though, that Dad used meat in extreme moderation. And remember, too, that Mom was a lacto-ovo vegetarian, like virtually all the vegetarians in my extended family. Both Mom and Dad used milk and butter and cream and eggs, which are animal products.

Who's to say what might have happened if both of them had abstained from animal products of all kinds? Perhaps it still would have ended in a tie, but it might have come a bit longer down the line.

Of course, living a long time isn't a contest, and we can be thankful for that. Who needs the pressure? Our goal simply is to be as healthy and happy as possible, each day, for the rest of our lives. And we should do whatever it takes to make that happen. If we do it right, our lives are more likely to be long ones. And happy ones.

Even though I cheat a little bit, and eat that occasional slice of pizza, or that rare Big Mac, or that once-in-a-blue-moon seafood dinner, I call myself a vegan these days, and I stand tall as I say it.

Dr. T. Colin Campbell, the director of the China Study, is stricter than I am. He refuses to call himself a vegan, even though he really is. It's because of his own little cheating episodes. Tiny, really.

In a 2009 interview with Charles Platkin, creator of the "Diet Detective" column, Campbell admitted that when his "wife isn't looking," he sometimes will eat a bit of "strongly flavored cheese." Never at home, of course. "It has to be someplace else, because it is not to be found in our house," he said.

He told the *New York Times* in 2011, "I don't use the word 'vegan' or 'vegetarian.' I don't like those words. I want people to talk about plant-based nutrition and to think about these ideas in a very empirical scientific sense, and not with an ideological bent to it. I'm talking about whole, plant-based foods. The effect it produces is broad for treatment and prevention of a wide variety of ailments, from cancer to heart disease to diabetes. It's not a religion with me, it's just that the closer we get to a 100 percent plant-based diet, the better off we're going to be."

Ellen G. White, my great-great-grandmother, became a world-famous vegetarian, but she grew up eating meat. She was sickly in her youth, even an invalid for periods of time, and her family believed that meat would help strengthen her. Indeed, flesh foods were her "principal article of diet," she later would recall. "I was a great meat eater."

In fact, she still was eating meat when she began her ministry. She was quite fond of meat, and it was not her idea to stop it. It was God's, she said.

She received a "great light from the Lord," she said, during a vision on June 6, 1863. She was informed that health and diet reform were to be an intrinsic part of the Adventist message. "I did not seek this light," she later reported. "I did not study to obtain it; it was given to me by the Lord to give to others. The Lord presented a general plan before me. I was shown that God would give to His commandment-keeping people a reform diet, and that as they received this, their disease and suffering would be greatly lessened" (*Counsels on Diet and Foods*, 1938).

She started to preach health reform immediately and with great passion. "Shall human beings live on the flesh of dead animals? The answer, from the light God has given, is No, decidedly No. Many die of diseases wholly due to meat eating. The intellectual, the moral, and the physical powers are depreciated by the habitual use of flesh meats. Meat eating deranges the system, beclouds the intellect, and blunts the moral sensibilities. We say to you, dear brother and sister, your safest course is to let meat alone. We have plenty of good things to satisfy hunger without bringing corpses upon our table to compose our bill of fare" (*Counsels on Diet and Foods*).

Though she spoke firmly, it's important to note that she never played the role of tyrant on the subject. She understood that reform is a transition, a process, a journey with checkpoints, twists and turns, starts and stops and restarts.

In urging Adventist missionaries to take the new health message to the world, she advised restraint and tact. She cautioned against pushing too hard, too fast, especially among populations that for generations had subsisted largely on flesh foods. In a letter of 1896, she wrote, "There should be no rash movements. We should consider the situation of the people, and the power of lifelong habits and practices . . . All should have the light in this question, but let it be carefully presented. Habits that have been thought right for a lifetime are not to be changed by harsh or hasty measures."

The early Adventists were declaring a new health message not only to the world, but also among themselves. And many of them found personal reform to be a challenge, not only as it applied to flesh foods but also to other indulgences. One story often told in my family concerns a pioneer church member named William Farnsworth, of Washington, New Hampshire. He tried valiantly to kick his tobacco habit after Ellen

G. White began preaching that tobacco is a "malignant poison." Alas, he had relapsed in the winter of 1867, and his nineteen-year-old son, Eugene, knew it. Father and son were working on their snow-covered property and Eugene could see that his dad was chewing tobacco and spitting into the snow. The elder Farnsworth tried to be discreet about it, even using his boot to kick snow over the stains. But the young Farnsworth was not to be fooled.

In December of that year, Ellen G. White visited the congregation and preached for five hours, urging believers to reaffirm their faith. She even shared what she said were direct admonitions from God to specific members of the audience. Young Eugene Farnsworth looked nervously at his father, wondering if God had told Sister White about those stains in the snow. He was stunned when, at that very moment, Ellen G. White turned and pointed directly to William Farnsworth and said, "I saw that this brother is a slave to tobacco."

She went on, admonishing him as much for his cover-up of the deed as for the deed itself. "But the worst of the matter," she said, "is that he is acting the part of a hypocrite, trying to deceive his brethren into thinking that he has discarded it, as he promised to do."

The moment had a double impact. Not only was William Farnsworth properly reproved, but also son Eugene Farnsworth, convinced beyond doubt that Ellen G. White was the true messenger of God, repurposed his life and became one of the church's great early evangelists, preaching the gospel for more than six decades in nations throughout the world. He also wrote a booklet titled "Divine Healing." He died in 1935 at the age of eighty-eight.

It must be said that health reform was a personal challenge for Ellen G. White, too. She continued to use meat on occasion, even long after she began preaching against it in principle. Sometimes, she used it out of necessity, when traveling or visiting in places where other options were not sufficiently available. "When I could not obtain the food I needed, I have sometimes eaten a little meat," she once said, "but I am becoming more and more afraid of it" (*Christian Temperance and Bible Hygiene*, 1890).

Sometimes, she would eat a little flesh food for no other reason, apparently, than she wanted to do so. In a letter of May 31, 1882, to her daughter-in-law Mary Kelsey White, the wife of her son Willie, she talked about her upcoming visit to their home in Oakland, California, and made a wish list of groceries she hoped her hosts could procure for her. "If you can get a good box of herrings—fresh ones—please do so. The last ones that Willie got are bitter and old. If you can get a few cans of good oysters, get them," she wrote.

As one might expect, her critics and detractors, then and now, have jumped all over anecdotes such as these to lambast Ellen G. White as a hypocrite. She was a liar, they say.

She cheated.

Well, say what they will about that, there's no gainsaying the vital fact that my great-great-grandmother accomplished two remarkable things as a health reformer. She took charge of her own body, which originally was weak and infirm, and transformed it into a physical dynamo that worked tirelessly for eighty-seven years, at a time when the average life expectancy was half of that. Also, she used the power of her ministry to create a whole global demographic that has grown to become one of the largest united vegetarian populations on Earth, the members of which are known for their health, fitness, and longevity.

She thought of health reform as a message of deliverance, not damnation. She was the bearer of good news, not bad news. She was no tyrant.

"Those who understand the laws of health and who are governed by principle," she said, "will shun the extremes, both of indulgence and restrictions. There is real common sense in dietetic reform. The subject should be studied broadly and deeply, and no one should criticize others because their practice is not, in all things, in harmony with his own. It is impossible to make an unvarying rule to regulate everyone's habits, and no one should think himself a criterion for all" (*Ministry of Healing*, 1905).

My late "Auntie" Grace, a granddaughter of Ellen G. White (and sister of my grandfather), told many stories about congenial family get-togethers at her grandmother's house. Meals were fun, she always remembered. The mood was merry, not morose. The idea was to eat well and feel good and be happy. (By the way, I will share secret family recipes with you before we are done!)

As a consequence of growing into her teens while Ellen G. White was still alive, and knowing her so well, Grace White Jacques grew up to share her grandmother's practical, commonsense attitudes about health and diet. Here's what she said in a 1978 interview with Dr. Patricia B. Mutch at a workshop titled "Ellen G. White and Dietetics" at Andrews University in Berrien Springs, Michigan: "Now it would be a great hardship for me to eat meat, but I wouldn't be that extreme. If I were in Alaska, or the South Sea Islands, and I couldn't get other food, I would eat what they had, because what is health reform but eating the best food available? We have so many things in this land. We don't have to eat things that are not best for us. I'm so grateful and I'm so thankful for the knowledge of healthful living. Now, we've always tried to live up to it. I wouldn't say we have done it a hundred percent, no one does that, you know, but I've tried all my life. I've been brought up on a healthful diet and I'm grateful, I'm thankful, and I think I can do a lot of things people my age can't do."

My "Auntie" Grace was seventy-eight when she spoke these words, and she would live another seventeen years!

How true it was for her to say, "We have so many things in this land." And it is even more true today than it was in 1978. Now, eating the world's best diet is far easier than it was generations, decades, even a few years ago. Improved methods of food production and transportation have resulted in a world where fresh fruits and vegetables of every kind are available everywhere on a year-round basis. New plant-based dairy alternatives and meat substitutes have come onto the market. Ancient grains, heirloom tomatoes, exotic legumes, "super fruits," and other interesting delicacies can be found in our produce aisles.

Friends, take advantage! Take the path to better health and longer life.

If you encounter a little bump along the way, deal with it and move past it. If temptation causes a little divergence in your direction, make it as short a detour as possible, stay out of the ditch, and get right back on the high road.

Ellen G. White herself may have cheated on her diet now and then, but she surely didn't get cheated out of the ultimate prize of long life and lasting accomplishments.

Take courage in this message, and take comfort in this promise. If Ellen G. White could cheat, if William Farnsworth could suffer a little relapse, if "Auntie" Grace could consider even the possibility of cheating, if my dad could cheat, if Uncle Floyd could cheat, if Dr. T. Colin Campbell can cheat, and if I myself can cheat, every once in a great while, you can cheat, too.

I won't tell.

As long as you cheat responsibly. And in moderation.

A Happy Home Remedy for Cheese Envy

I have many vegetarian friends who can't quite pull the trigger on going vegan. It's not because they're hooked on dairy products in general. No, it's because they're hooked on one dairy product in particular. Listen to a conversation I had with a friend just last weekend:

> **HER:** I would miss cheese.
>
> **ME:** Don't make a face at me, but have you tried the nut cheeses, the soy cheeses, the rice cheeses?
>
> **HER** (making a face): I can't find those.
>
> **ME:** They're everywhere! You'll find a few in most grocery stores, and you'll find a lot more in health food stores. Cheddar, jack, mozzarella . . . all the flavors. They come in blocks, slices, shredded . . . whatever you want.
>
> **HER** (making a face): They don't taste the same.
>
> **ME:** OK, if you eat them by themselves, you'll notice a difference. But in a sandwich, or a veggie taco, or a casserole, they get the job done. They're melty, gooey, stretchy . . . just like cheese!
>
> **HER** (making a face): What about pizza? Pizza IS cheese!
>
> **ME:** No way. You'll find cheeseless pizza as a menu item at lots of restaurants, even pizza parlors. Or make your own. Pizza bread, tomato sauce, shredded

mozzarella or jack cheese substitute, loads of mushrooms, onions, olives, chile peppers, whatever. Bake for ten minutes at 500 degrees. Boom. Done. You'll love it!

HER (making a face): I don't know. I would miss regular pizza.

ME: OK, have a slice of regular pizza now and then.

HER (brightening): Really?

ME: Go ahead. If an occasional slice of regular pizza helps you maintain an otherwise dairy-free diet, you definitely are coming out ahead.

HER: Isn't that cheating?

ME: You know what? You're going to enjoy one of the chapters in my new book. It's a chapter called "Cheating in Moderation."

CHAPTER SIX

The Fundamentals
of Supplementals

I LOVE BROWSING IN HEALTH FOOD STORES.

I know. Weird, huh?

Turn me loose in one of those, and I'm like a kid in a candy shop.

I dig the good smells in there. Yeasty, earthy, vital smells. Whole grains and garden greens. Seeds and sprouts. Beans and nuts.

I love the sights in there, too. So many colors, so many interesting shapes, so many varieties of things. Big bins full of barley and bulgur and buckwheat. Crunchy cereals by the bag. Bright fruits and vegetables fresh from the field.

There's always something new. Milk made from cashews! Sausage made from mushrooms! What will they come up with next?

I've been browsing in health food stores for my entire life. My Aunt Kay and Uncle Barney Matheson were pioneers in the business. They founded Full O' Life Natural Foods Market and Restaurant more than fifty years ago in beautiful downtown Burbank.

And as mentioned earlier, I grew up just an hour away, in Loma Linda, where there is another trailblazing health food store, the Loma Linda Market, established in the 1930s.

So, you see, I'm a bit of an expert on the subject of health food stores, and I've noticed two big changes over the course of many decades, at least here in Southern California where I live.

First, there are many, many more of these stores than there used to be. And, second, there has been a major shift in what they sell.

When I was a kid, health food stores were more like grocery stores. They sold mostly food. They also sold vitamin, mineral, and herbal supplements, but these usually were confined to a shelf or two in a corner of the store.

Today, in a great number of health food stores, it's the other way around. The supplements have taken over the place. They're in the front and middle, where they can't be missed. Vitamins and minerals and herbs by the thousands, in bottles and jars and boxes and bags, stocked on shelf after shelf, in aisle after aisle. It's the fresh produce and other grocery items that are in the corners now. They've been squeezed to the perimeter, pushed to the side, to make room for all the supplements.

There are even stores, nowadays, that have done away with food altogether. Vitamins and minerals are all they sell. Pills, powders, and potions of every kind.

More than half of adult Americans (53 percent) take supplements, according to a 2011 report by the U.S. Centers for Disease Control and Prevention. The Consumer Reports organization says the supplement industry has boomed in the last twenty-five years to become a $27 billion giant.

That's a lot of money.

Out of curiosity, I visited one of the big chain health food stores near where I live, and I started doing the math as I explored the supplement aisles. Theoretically, how much would it cost me to buy one each of everything?

I didn't get very far. I only made it down a fraction of one half of one aisle before I realized I would need a supercomputer in my head for this experiment. The dollar amount would be gigantic. It would be a figure too huge for my brain to manage. My wallet was getting nervous, too, even though this was purely an information-gathering exercise and not a spending spree.

I decided to try something a bit more practical. I visited my nearest Costco warehouse store, which has a big supplement department but carries only the basic, most popular, best-selling essentials. That's what Costco does, masterfully. It edits everything down to a few easy choices. You don't have to comparison shop between dozens of different brands of, say, ginkgo biloba (an herb taken for alertness and memory support). Costco has done it for you!

Here, I was able to conduct my experiment quite efficiently, though admittedly I still ended up with a case of sticker shock. I roamed up and down each aisle, keeping a mental tab of the price of everything from astaxanthin (for healthy skin) to zinc (for immune support).

I calculated that if I were to buy only one container of only one brand of each vitamin, mineral, and herbal supplement in the store, my bill would come to more than $700.

Yes, my eyes widened a bit, and I might have gulped once or twice, but I was in no danger of actually spending that kind of loot on that stuff.

But there are people who do. Millions of them. They go into stores that sell supplements and they spend hundreds, even thousands, of dollars.

Why?

Is it because they are health conscious, and already eating right, and exercising well, and they want to take pills as extra insurance to bolster their continuing perfect health?

I don't think so. I suspect that in most cases these are people who are not eating right, and not exercising well, and they're popping pills as a substitute for what they should be doing.

That's right—they're not supplementing, they're substituting! They won't take care of themselves, so they're hoping that magic pills and potions will do it for them.

Good luck with that.

Here's a better idea. Start eating the world's best diet, consisting of plant-based whole foods, and you will not need to worry about vitamins and minerals. You're covered. You're supplied. You don't need extras. You don't need supplements.

Here's what our hero, Dr. T. Colin Campbell, director of the China Study, has to say on this subject: "There now is ample evidence that, except perhaps for B12 and maybe vitamin D, taking vitamin supplements is, at minimum, a waste of money and, at worst, may actually cause harm."

Wow, how about that! Dr. Campbell and I have just saved you hundreds of dollars! Maybe even thousands, depending on where you buy your supplements, and how many of them you buy, and how often.

But wait a minute. I don't exactly want everyone to stop buying vitamins and minerals and herbs right now. Remember, I was reared around health food stores, and there always were jars and bottles of vitamins and minerals around the house. There are two I remember most fondly. One was vitamin C, which we all would start gobbling whenever we felt a cold coming on. Mind you, this was decades before Nobel Prize–winning chemist Linus Pauling popularized the idea in his 1970 book *Vitamin C and the Common Cold*. I have no idea why it took him so long to discover what my family had known forever! (I'll have more to say about this in a later chapter, titled "Cure for the Common Cold.")

My other favorite was vitamin E, which I admired more for its looks than its purpose. Those luminous golden orbs! I used to stare at the clear glass jar of them, and move the jar around in the sunlight to make the capsules gleam, then tilt the jar to make them roll and tumble like cascading jewels! It was mesmerizing.

I know. Weird, huh?

By the way, Dr. T. Colin Campbell doesn't want you to stop taking supplements, either. Not all of them, anyway. Study his words again. He gives vitamin D a thumbs-up. And he gives vitamin B12 an even bigger thumbs-up.

Here's the thing about vitamin B12, which benefits your brain and nervous system. It's the only nutrient of its kind that is not abundantly supplied by a vegan diet. The way I have heard it explained is that plant foods once were rich with B12 but modern farming methods have over-worked and stripped the soil of that vitamin.

Boy, oh boy, my grandfather would have had plenty to say about that!

Herbert C. White was a pioneer organic gardener who already was composting soil in the 1940s and then writing about it in the 1950s. He served as garden editor of *Let's Live* magazine, a popular national health and fitness magazine. And one of the books he coauthored with Dr. H. E. Kirschner, *Are You What You Eat?* (1960), deals extensively with soil husbandry. He was of the zealous opinion that mankind was threatening itself with extinction through improper farming methods, soil neglect, and the use of pesticides.

He wrote, "It is a sad fact that our U.S. soils are becoming more and more deficient in minerals, and less and less fertile . . . What a trag-edy that the majority of American farmers still condone practices that inhibit and destroy the LIVING soil. When will farmers WAKE UP to the FACTS OF LIFE? It's later than we think!"

That's my grandfather for you. Lots of capital letters and exclama-tion points.

And, in the same way that I now am writing about him in my book, he wrote about his grandmother in his book. Listen to him:

"For some seven years, as young lads, my twin brother Henry and I were privileged to act as helpers on Ellen G. White's beautiful Napa Valley ranch in northern California. By the way, this grandmother of ours was a confirmed organic gardener. No chemical fertilizers were ever permitted on the Elmshaven dairy and fruit farm; and what is more, to my knowledge no poison sprays were ever used in the orchards or vegetable gardens. She always believed in cooperating with Nature instead of fighting her."

One of the chapters in *Are You What You Eat?* is titled "How I Treat a Sick Tree." My grandfather tells the story of how he saved an apple tree by correcting and feeding the soil around its roots. He undertook the challenge as a demonstration project for a series of classes he was teaching in 1954 in Washington, D.C.

The chapter includes "before" and "after" pictures. The tree looks scrawny and pathetic in the first photo, but in the second it is blooming in full glory, and there's a beautiful woman standing next to it. My grandfather's caption reads, "Our photograph shows my daughter Dorothy standing by the little tree just one year after treatment."

Hey, that's my mom!

OK, that's enough of a detour down memory lane for now. Let's get back to the subject of vitamins and minerals.

A vitamin B12 supplement is a smart choice for anyone, and a necessary choice for vegans. Having some vitamin D supplements around the house is a good idea, too. But trust me, if you're eating right, your normal needs for most vitamins and minerals are supplied in full. You can stop worrying about whether you're getting enough of this or enough of that. You don't need to pop a lot of extra pills.

Now, if taking a simple multivitamin every day gives you a little shot of psychological insurance, by all means go ahead. It's no worse than Popeye downing that extra can of spinach when he wants a boost. He obviously doesn't need it, considering the fact that he eats spinach all the time, but there's no harm in it, so why not? (Hopefully, he also is eating lots of other good veggies and fruits and nuts and whole grains to go with those greens!)

Here's one more word of caution, though, on the subject of supplements. There are some that actually have been red-flagged as potentially dangerous, so you don't want to be carefree about taking those. You see, the supplement industry is not federally regulated like the pharmaceutical industry. Products are not tested and product claims are not checked with the same level of oversight. This is a sore point for the Consumer Reports organization and other watchdog groups.

"There's a false perception that supplements fall under the same regulatory umbrella as prescription drugs," said Dr. Orly Avitzur, medical adviser for *Consumer Reports*, quoted in a 2011 CNN report. "That's not the case. We really don't know what's inside."

That's why consumers are urged to take a buyer-beware approach to supplements, especially those few that have caused alarm about their potential adverse side effects or unsafe interactions with prescription medications. Some such supplements have even appeared on the radar of the U.S. Food and Drug Administration, which usually pays little attention to the industry.

Colloidal silver, for example, a mineral used by some people for immune support and protection against infection, can cause permanent skin discoloration, according to the FDA, which started warning against the supplement in October 2009. Unless you want to start looking like one of the blue aliens in the movie *Avatar*, you better be careful with that one.

Kava, an herb used by some to treat anxiety, has been linked to liver damage. It is banned in Canada and some European countries.

Lobelia, used for respiratory support, can cause unsafe changes in heartbeat and blood pressure, according to the FDA, which started warning against the herb in 1993.

Comfrey, used for centuries all over the world to treat a wide range of skin and internal disorders, has been linked in recent years with liver damage and cancer. The FDA took the unusual step of banning its sale for internal use starting in July 2001.

My grandfather REALLY would have jumped up and down and had something to say about that one! He was a big believer in the benefits of comfrey. In another of the books he co-wrote with Dr. H. E. Kirschner, *Nature's Healing Grasses* (1960), comfrey appears in the starring role. One chapter is titled "Comfrey—The Healer," another is titled "Comfrey—The Miracle Herb," and a third is titled "A Leaf a Day Keeps Illness Away."

Yikes!

We all know that conventional wisdom undergoes change over time. Information gets updated.

The best idea, as in all cases, is to use common sense when it comes to buying and using nutritional and dietary supplements. If you see a vitamin, mineral, or herbal supplement that is touted as a miracle cure for anything (or everything), be afraid, be very afraid. If it's some pill or potion about which you know nothing, get some expert advice before you waste your good money and possibly your good health.

If you're looking at the basic vitamins named after the first few letters of the alphabet, go ahead, you are probably in the clear. But if you're looking at vitamins named after other letters of the alphabet, please report their existence immediately to health science authorities, who so far possess no knowledge of them.

Of course, that may change. As the supplement industry continues to grow and expand, we probably one day can expect to see vitamins named after every letter of the alphabet.

Vitamin Z, anyone? Yes, it protects you from zombie bites!

Yeah, right.

Remember this, above all else: Supplements are not substitutes for sound health practices.

"It's a Band-Aid approach to think you can eat poorly and just take a vitamin and you'll be equal to another person who eats well and exercises and takes care of their health and gets regular checkups," said Dr. Avitzur, the *Consumer Reports* medical adviser, quoted by CNN. "There's no substitute for a healthy lifestyle."

I asked my brother Doug, the doctor, if he takes supplements. He told me he takes six, faithfully, every day: vitamin B-complex, vitamin C, vitamin D, vitamin E, a basic multivitamin, and zinc.

Now, let me visit my kitchen and see what's on my own pill shelf. Yes, I have a pill shelf.

Hmm, right now I have saw palmetto (prostate health support), potassium (heart and kidneys), calcium (bones), vitamin B-complex (which includes vitamin B12), vitamin C, vitamin E, zinc and echinacea (both for immune support), a "green drink" powder mix, a new thing called garcinia cambogia (an exotic fruit extract in capsule form that is touted as a fat blocker), and some omega-3 fish oil.

Fish oil? That's an old one. I didn't know I still had it around. I need to throw it out and replace it with some good vegan flaxseed oil!

(I checked with my cousin-in-law, Clint Comstock, who is the vitamins and minerals expert at Full O' Life Natural Foods in Burbank, and he said it was OK to make the switch. Fish oil is still his first choice, though.)

Here's the thing with me. I don't take any of this stuff every day. That's why there are inconsistencies, even incongruities, to be found on my pill shelf. Why is there no vitamin D, for example, when there are all those other vitamins? Why is there crazy stuff like garcinia cambogia? Why is there old stuff like fish oil, which I don't take at all anymore?

I'm not like my brother Doug, the doctor, who is consistent and wise. Obviously, he got the brains between the two of us.

Seriously, though, vitamin and mineral supplements are hit and miss with me. Mostly miss.

And that's OK.

Like I said, all the vitamins and minerals our bodies need are adequately supplied by the foods we should be eating. And I definitely am not hit and miss about the foods I eat. No, I try never to miss a good meal!

But days, weeks, even months will go by and most of my pill shelf will go untouched. Then, on a whim, I'll start taking one of everything, every day, for a while. Or maybe one of this and one of that. Every day. For a while.

And, if I hear about some new amazing thing on TV like garcinia cambogia, I'll run out and buy a jar and try that every day. For a while. Then forget about it.

I guess I like having a few supplements around. It's the way I grew up. So, I buy them. I have them. I just hardly ever take them.

I know. Weird, huh?

A Happy Home Remedy for Vitamin B12 Deficiency

Look for foods that say they are fortified with vitamin B12, including some nondairy milk products, some meat substitute products, and some breakfast cereals. Also, take a vitamin B12 supplement each day. It's the best way to ensure that you're getting enough. Fortunately, it's easy to do. Vitamin B12 is available on its own, or in combination with other B vitamins in most vitamin B-complex supplements. It's also available in sufficient amounts in most multivitamin supplements. Some people are better able to absorb vitamin B12 if they take the supplements in chewable form. These are widely available. Finally, vitamin B12 loses potency if exposed to sunlight, so store your vitamin B12 (and other supplements) in a cool, dry, dark place.

CHAPTER SEVEN

A Resounding
Chorus of Booze

I'VE HEARD IT ON GOOD AUTHORITY—FROM DOCTORS, EVEN—THAT DRINKING A couple of glasses of red wine each day will add years to my life. This is good news. At the rate I go through red wine, I should live approximately forever!

Ha ha ha! I am kidding, of course.

Actually, I'm not kidding, but I do know better.

I do know that just because a little wine is good for us does not mean that a lot of wine is even better.

Darn it. It's that whole moderation thing again.

I get so bored with moderation sometimes. Why couldn't we have ended up on a planet where moderation is bad, and it's excess that is good for us?

Maybe heaven is like that. Champagne mimosas for breakfast, beers at lunch, wine at dinner, and tequila shots all night. Party on!

I know. I'm dreaming.

Booze was very taboo in my family. My mother came from a long line of crusading abstainers, and there was a bona fide drunkard or two in my father's lineage. Believe me, alcohol can be just as unpopular among the descendants of boozers as among the descendants of teetotalers.

I think I even was spanked once, as a child, after I spontaneously erupted into a spirited song rendition of one of the popular beer jingles of the day: "National Beer! National Beer! You'll love the taste of National Beer! And while I'm about it I'm proud to say, it's brewed on the shores of the Chesapeake Bay!"

Alcohol was so forbidden, so condemned, so cloaked in ignominy in my family that I, of course, found it deeply fascinating. That's the kind of curious little bugger I was. I wanted to know more, not less, about mysteries such as this. I was drawn by temptation to alcohol as surely as the moth is drawn by temptation to the candle flame.

I had my first drink when I was nine or ten.

Well, it wasn't a drink, really. It was more like a tiny sip. OK, a lot of tiny sips.

My pal Jay, who also was nine or ten, would go walking with me along Adelphi Road, which in those days was pretty rural, with lots of wooded areas on both sides. Motorists always felt carefree about flinging out their empty beer, wine, and liquor bottles there. As a consequence, there always was a fresh supply of new bottles each day, and a fair number of them would have a trickle or two of drink still in them.

I use the word "fresh" with some hesitation because there is nothing even remotely fresh about the flavor of old booze, baked hot in the sunshine, and probably with a little bit of somebody's spit mixed into it.

But this is what we settled for, young Jay and I, as our introduction into the sophisticated world of adult beverages. The beer tasted terrible, but we strained for each drop. Wine was even worse, sour and sticky, but we let nothing go to waste. Our favorite was whiskey, which had deeper, darker, more concentrated flavors. Sometimes we would find several whiskey bottles and combine the drops from all of them into one bottle, so each of us could get something close to a whole swallow's worth of liquor. Old Crow was the brand we found most often, so it must have been the local crowd favorite at the time. Or maybe it was just the choice of one guy who did a whole lot of drinking and driving on Adelphi Road.

Shame on him.

And shame on us, too. What brats we were!

I don't recall that we ever got tipsy as a result of those salvage operations. The volume for that just wasn't there.

So, it's not like we became hardened alcoholics at the age of nine or ten.

In fact, once those boyish adventures played themselves out, there was no more alcohol for me until college days, other than the occasional shenanigans that high school students pull.

I will confess, though, that once I was off to college I wasted no time in becoming a man of cosmopolitan thirst. For years I drank mostly beer, because that's what college students do. And it was good beer, by the way. Today's beer-flavored water drinks known as "lite" beers had not yet been invented, thankfully.

Then, a few years out of college, I became fond of fine wine. I remember the day it happened, in fact. My hiking companion and I stood in the woods near Forest Falls in the San Bernardino Mountains. A light snow started to fall, so we decided to call it a day and head back down to the car. First, though, we opened and shared a bottle of wine I had brought along. It was an expensive Napa Valley cabernet sauvignon. I think someone had given it to me as a gift.

This was a complex red wine, far different from the lightweight wines with which we were more familiar, being infrequent wine drinkers. At first taste, we grimaced. But the snow kept falling, gently, and the wine produced a warming effect, and we handed the bottle back and forth with increasing rapidity. By the time it was half gone, we agreed it was not too bad. By the time it was three-quarters spent, we declared it to be excellent. By the time it was all gone, we had become confirmed oenophiles for life.

For years I remained fully satisfied as a partaker of wine and beer only, but eventually my drinking career came full circle, and I again started to sample the blandishments of whiskey and other spirited liquors, as I had done on a very small scale as a very small boy. Of course, I now wasn't drinking just the last drops of a bottle I had found along the roadside, but all the drops in a bottle I had purchased at the store.

I look back with some ruefulness on this development because hard liquor is about three times as strong as wine, just as wine is about twice as strong as beer, so there is an obvious escalation of risk factors that comes into play here. Great care must be taken. The need for moderation becomes more and more important as one contends with stronger and stronger forces.

Believe me, these are what are called "lessons learned" for me, and I don't share them with you lightly.

Alcohol can be a mighty foe if mistreated, just as it can be a steady friend if treated well.

I always have tried my best to get along amicably with it, but sometimes I have overplayed my hand. Alcohol pairs well with my questing nature, my sense of adventure, my curiosity about what marvels are to be seen around the next bend, but, alas, alcohol and I don't always travel well together. We have our ups and downs. It's a complicated relationship.

I wish I wasn't quite so fond it.

But, honestly, is there a refreshment in all of creation that is so beguiling, so seductive, so affectionate toward so many of our senses?

That is why we must be so wary of its wiles, so cautious in our entanglements with it.

There is no other elixir than alcohol that is available in so many flavors for our tongues to taste, and so many colors for our eyes to admire, and so many fragrances for our noses to savor. Even our ears are delighted by the fizz of sparkling wines, or the whisper of beer as it foams in the glass, or the tumbling of ice cubes as we stir a cocktail. And our sense of touch is aroused when we lift the glass to drink and feel the heft in our hands and the tingle on our lips.

And what other elixir comes in bottles of so many enchanting shapes and tints? Even rainbows are not more beautiful than a row of spirit bottles that gleam upon a shelf in front of a light.

And what other elixir fascinates not only our bodily senses but our minds and emotions, too, calling to us with a longing siren song, giving form to our dreams, quickening our imaginations, inviting us and urging us to undertake brave exploits in strange faraway places?

What other elixir excites our ambitions, calms our doubts, forgives our faults, redresses our past mistakes, assures us that we can be great poets, great champions, or great lovers, and then charms us into taking the chance?

OK, that's probably enough rhapsodizing about booze. This is a health book, for crying out loud.

Drinking too much is unhealthy, and many millions of people cannot resist the temptation to drink too much. Alcohol is addicting, quite literally as well as figuratively. It is a substance that begs for abuse, and it never lacks for volunteers. It commands a slave army of abusers who themselves become the abused.

There are very few choices, and very few outcomes, for addicts.

Some alcoholics succumb to their affliction and ruin their lives. Often, they ruin the lives of others, as well.

Some alcoholics save themselves by pulling back totally from alcohol's clutching embrace and renouncing it completely and forever.

It's not easy.

One famous success story involves a friend and hero of mine, the great writer James Brown who lives in Lake Arrowhead, less than a half hour's drive up the hill from where I live.

I call him my drinking buddy, but not because we drink together. No way. That's never going to happen.

He's not drinking these days, you see.

But he used to drink, big time, and I call him my drinking buddy because that's what we talk about whenever we get together. Drinking. That's right, we talk about drinking.

"Alcoholism and drug addiction are my favorite topics," Brown says cheerfully. "There's nothing I'd rather talk about."

Brown not only talks about drinking. He writes about drinking. *The Los Angeles Diaries*, which won numerous literary prizes when it appeared in 2003, is Brown's unsparing memoir of how his dysfunctional family, which included an abusive mother who spent time in prison, and two siblings who committed suicide, sent his own life on the skids. He became a manic-depressive bully, a drunk, and a junkie.

A sequel, *This River* (2011), tells how his depression and addictions plagued him as he attempted to build his own family and career. It was rough going.

Brown writes with brutal force and frankness about the epic battles between his demons and himself. I will urge anyone who is teetering on the brink of addiction, or fighting in the trenches with it, to please buy and read *This River*. Two chapters in particular, "Instructions on the Use of Alcohol" and "Instructions on the Use of Heroin," surely are among the most harrowing indictments against those two indulgences ever rendered into words.

Brown quit drinking and drugging quite a few years ago. He promises to describe his recovery in a third memoir that will complete the trilogy of his story and put a happy ending on it. Whew! That will be a relief!

Brown quit substance abuse because he had to quit. It was do or die. He absolutely made the right choice, and I am glad he did it.

I would hate to lose my drinking buddy.

Now, myself, I'm not ready to quit drinking. I don't want to quit. At least not completely. I believe that a truly moderate amount of drinking is good for us. And I take pleasure in reminding everyone that booze is vegan. Unless, of course, you wreck it by making those wretched milky or eggnoggy drinks. No thanks!

If I ever do decide it is time to quit drinking altogether, I will do it. And I'll let you know how it goes. And, by the way, I won't do it cold turkey. That can shock the system and cause stroke or heart attack. It's true. It has happened to people I know.

No, quitting should be done just like drinking should be done. In measured increments. That's right, quitting should be done in moderation. Ironic, huh?

Like I said, I hope I don't have to come to that crossroads and make that decision. I hope I can continue to walk the semi-straight line that veers between drinking too much and drinking not at all.

For what it's worth, I have a few tips to offer on how to do that. And, believe me, these are battle-tested tips from the front lines.

First, follow doctors' orders and limit yourself to one or two drinks each day. Mind you, these drinks must be of conventional size. No fair filling up a fish bowl and calling it a glass. No, the serving sizes we are talking about are 12 ounces of beer, 5 ounces of wine, and 1.5 ounces of liquor.

Second, if a rare day comes when you find yourself tempted to imbibe in slightly more than one or two drinks, because you have been invited to a Kardashian wedding, let us say, and the champagne is exquisite, then pace yourself, please, by drinking a tall glass of water between each of the wicked drinks.

Third, don't ever drink on an empty stomach. Always drink with a meal. Preferably not breakfast. That just looks bad. Come on!

Most importantly, don't drink at all if you are about to do anything that is the slightest bit dangerous, such as driving, using sharp tools, or discussing politics with strangers.

If you hurt yourself, and possibly others, all of that good health for which you have been striving can be gone in an instant.

That's a sobering thought, isn't it?

A Happy Home Remedy for Hangover

Too much to drink? Shame on you. But let's get you back on your feet, so you can start walking the straight and narrow. That's what you're going to do, right?

Excess alcohol in your system leaves you dehydrated and depleted of nutrients. The blood vessels in your head are swollen, which causes headaches. You are suffering from acidosis, which means your blood is too acidic, which causes nausea and sweating.

First, drink water. Lots of water. Two 8-ounce glasses, at least. You need to rehydrate. You should have done this before you went to sleep (or passed out) last night. It would have helped. Now, you have some catching up to do.

Have a cup of coffee. Not too much. It's a diuretic, which will dehydrate you all over again. But one cup's worth will help constrict the dilated blood vessels in your head, which will ease your headache.

Have a little ginger. The chemical compound gingerol is an amazingly effective remedy against nausea. Chew a bit of peeled fresh ginger, or take ginger in capsule form (available at health food stores), or drink a strong cup of ginger tea (available in tea bags at health food stores). Even ginger candy or ginger ale are effective, as long as they contain real ginger and not just ginger flavoring.

Eat a little food. Leftover enchiladas would be good. Something substantial. Lasagna works, too. (And, by the way, you'll find terrific recipes for enchiladas and lasagna in chapter twenty-one of this book.) If nothing hearty is handy, at least have a slice of toast with jam. Better yet, have a slice of toast with Marmite, the yeast extract spread that is an obsession in Great Britain. It's as thick and black as hot asphalt, and about as pungent, but it's ridiculously rich in vitamins and minerals. Similarly obsessed Australians have their own version, called Vegemite, and there's an American version called Vegex. You'll find one or more brands in most health food stores. Warning: This is salty stuff, so take it easy. Spread it nice and thin. Double warning: You will find yourself joining one of two sides, those who love it dearly or those who loathe it bitterly. There is no middle ground.

CHAPTER EIGHT

The Other Buzz Drinks— Coffee, Tea, and Whee!

I ONCE HEARD BILLY GRAHAM SAY IN AN INTERVIEW THAT, YES, HE DID HAVE ONE vice. "I drink coffee, and I would find it hard to give it up," the famed evangelist confessed.

This taught me two things.

First, I now believe he is the most righteous man of all time, if coffee is the only blemish on his record. Second, it taught me that Baptists, at least some of them like Billy Graham, are at least a little bit wary of coffee and regard it as something of a guilty pleasure.

This was interesting to me because the Seventh-day Adventist church also looks askance at coffee. And tea. And caffeinated soft drinks.

In fact, the Adventists are way tougher than the Baptists.

I enjoy driving over to California Baptist University in Riverside, not far from where I live, for the occasional lunch in the excellent campus cafeteria there. Not only is the food great, but I also can get a cup of good strong coffee, too, if I want it. Or tea. Or caffeinated soft drinks.

These beverages are not available in the cafeteria on the campus of Loma Linda University, where I also go for lunch now and then. I can get an excellent vegetarian meal there, and perhaps a cup of decaf coffee, or herbal tea, or a caffeine-free soft drink, but if it's caffeine I crave, I am better off hanging out with the Baptists.

Now, it's not like coffee is a deal breaker for the Adventists. It's not a test of fellowship. You can be an Adventist in good standing and drink all the coffee and tea and Coca-Cola you want, on your own, but institutionally it is not served. You won't find it in Adventist cafeterias or in the social halls of Adventist churches or any place where Adventists gather officially as a group.

You see, Ellen G. White would not approve.

"In relation to tea, coffee, tobacco, and alcoholic drinks, the only safe course is to touch not, taste not, handle not," my great-great-grand-mother wrote in *Ministry of Healing* (1905). "It must be kept before the people that the right balance of the mental and moral powers depends in a great degree on the right condition of the physical system. All narcotics and unnatural stimulants that enfeeble and degrade the physical nature tend to lower the tone of the intellect and morals. Intemperance lies at the foundation of the moral depravity of the world. By the indulgence of perverted appetite, man loses his power to resist temptation."

There are numerous other faith organizations that also frown on coffee and other stimulating drinks. The Mormons, for example, are as strict as, if not stricter than, the Adventists.

Mormon founder Joseph Smith reported in 1833 that it was God's decision that tea and coffee are "not for the body or belly" of believers. Church leaders later added caffeinated soft drinks to the proscribed list, which is why root beer, not Coke, is the soda of choice for most Mormons.

Adventists are crazy about root beer, too, by the way.

Generally, the complaint of religion against coffee and similar beverages is that they stimulate people in a physical, temporal way instead of the spiritual way that is preferred. Believers are supposed to get buzzed in Bible class, not in coffee bars. They're supposed to get stirred up by the indwelling of the Holy Spirit, not jolted and jacked up by hot cups of java.

The Adventist position on the issue is a little more wide-ranging than that. Ellen G. White, characteristically, added a health angle to her admonition against caffeine drinks.

"The habit of drinking tea and coffee is a greater evil than is often suspected," she wrote in *Christian Temperance and Bible Hygiene* (1890). "Many who have accustomed themselves to the use of stimulating drinks, suffer from headache and nervous prostration, and lose much time on account of sickness. They imagine they cannot live without the stimulus, and are ignorant of its effect upon health. What makes it the more dangerous is that its evil effects are so often attributed to other causes.

"Through the use of stimulants, the whole system suffers. The nerves are unbalanced, the liver is morbid in its action, the quality and circulation of the blood are affected, and the skin becomes inactive and sallow. The mind, too, is injured. The immediate influence of these stimulants is to excite the brain to undue activity, only to leave it weaker and less capable of exertion."

There never was coffee, tea, or caffeinated soda pop around the house while I was growing up. In fact, I got in big trouble once when my parents found an empty Coca-Cola can in the kitchen trash. I was the sole suspect, of course, being the oldest of their children and the only one with pocket money and a car. I was interrogated as if I had committed a capital crime.

Mind you, I was a senior in high school at the time. I was class president. I was an editor of both the campus newspaper and the yearbook. I was getting good grades. I was working a full-time job, too, and paying my own tuition. In fact, the Coke can in the wastebasket was the result, I'm sure, of the long hours I put in every day and night. I was a busy bee.

But, as proud of me as my parents usually may have been, and I think they were, my youthful achievements came to nothing during that one terrible moment when I was unmasked as nothing more than a hopped-up teenage Coke head.

It wasn't until I was married, and in a home of my own, that there was coffee and tea in the cupboard, and Coca-Cola in the fridge.

I remember my first wife and I had a few little parties, with some of our Adventist friends over, and we all would gather around the coffeepot and enthuse over it with absurd gusto. Oh, yes, we were flush-faced freedom fighters celebrating our glorious liberation!

Lo, these many years later, I still enjoy coffee and I would find it hard to give it up. I guess Billy Graham and I are a lot alike!

And, by the way, I take my coffee strong and black. That's right, I like coffee that actually tastes like coffee, not that awful milky, sugary, candy-flavored goop that today's so-called coffee lovers slurp in such great quantities at such high prices at so many oh-so-trendy establishments.

I proudly drink my unadulterated coffee, and I drink it every day. I also enjoy strong black tea, now and then, and the occasional Coke or Mountain Dew or one of the other caffeinated soft drinks.

However, I claim complete victory in my ongoing efforts to moderate my use of caffeine drinks. Caffeine is habit-forming but my habit is well under control, I am pleased to report, because a couple such drinks in a day is all I want or need. I almost always avoid them in the later afternoon or evening, for fear of disrupting my golden slumbers. As it happens, I enjoy Sanka or other decaf coffees, and even those roasted grain beverages such as Postum, Cafix, and Pero, and I dearly love all the flavorful herbal teas, so I find it very easy to switch to these caffeine-free alternatives when it's late in the day.

I never touch the so-called energy drinks. I tried them a couple of times and they made me feel as jumpy as a startled spider. I did not enjoy that feeling at all. I know some of these beverages contain no more caffeine than coffee, but some of them contain astronomically more, and the fact that most brands do not list caffeine amounts (the Food and Drug Administration does not require them to do so) makes me leery. I also don't like the fact that most of them are loaded with sugar. I am no fonder of diabetes, or tooth rot, than I am of jittery nerves.

Caffeine is a drug. It is a bitter crystalline compound extracted from coffee beans (hence, coffee), tea leaves (hence, tea), and kola nuts (hence, cola drinks). Nobody who ever has experienced that unpleasant "coffee headache," which often afflicts coffee drinkers when they fail to get their daily fix, can doubt the habituating effect of caffeine.

I rarely get headaches but, sure enough, when I do, I am puzzled at first until I realize that, oh, yes, I didn't have my morning coffee.

I suppose that means I am a little bit of an addict, after all. But I am coping well, so far, thank you very much.

Another clue in the case against the immoderate use of coffee and other caffeine drinks is the great number of coffee jokes and one-liners to be found in our pop culture, all of which point to our dependency on the stuff.

Drumroll, please! "A balanced diet consists of a cup of coffee in each hand!" LOL!

Drumroll! "INSTANT HUMAN: Just Add Coffee!" Ba da bing!

Drumroll! "I can't concentrate. There's too much blood in my caffeine stream!" Rim shot!

All joking aside, here's the real deal. Caffeine arouses pleasure centers in our brain and stimulates our nervous system, and you are right, it sounds very suspiciously fun. It's no wonder that people want to have it every day. And the fact that there's a historical record that documents many centuries of happy caffeine use by billions of people worldwide would seem to indicate that it's reasonably safe in moderation.

On the other hand, as it was foretold by my great-great-grandmother more than a hundred years ago, the immoderate use of caffeine has been linked scientifically to numerous physical afflictions, including nervous tremors, insomnia, dehydration, acid reflux, and diarrhea. In extreme cases there is risk of spiking blood pressure, irregular heartbeat, seizures, even death.

A U.S. Senate hearing was convened in 2013 after a Maryland teenager died of what an autopsy report described as "cardiac arrhythmia due to caffeine intoxication" after she had consumed two 24-ounce energy drinks. The senators also were responding to a report by the federal Substance Abuse and Mental Health Services Administration that the annual number of emergency room visits involving energy drinks had doubled to almost 21,000 between the years 2007 and 2011. About 1,500 of the cases involved children ages twelve to seventeen.

The senators called on the FDA to investigate the safety of energy drinks and also recommended an independent inquiry into the industry's marketing techniques, especially its advertising efforts aimed at young people.

One senator, Edward J. Markey of Massachusetts, a veteran of Capitol Hill's long campaign to curb smoking in public places and restrict tobacco advertising, said that today's energy drink manufacturers target youthful consumers in the same way that tobacco companies historically have done.

"Hook 'em early, keep 'em for life," Senator Markey said, sarcastically. "Makes a lot of sense to me as a marketing promotion."

Senator Richard J. Durbin of Illinois, another veteran of the congressional "tobacco wars," agreed. "It struck me that we were back into the same problem," he said, comparing the new concerns over energy drinks to the long-standing concerns over tobacco.

What should we make of it all?

Just this, and it applies as much to coffee, tea, and caffeinated soda pop as it does to energy drinks.

Be cool in your use of caffeine.

Also, consider this, please.

If you are eating a plant-based whole foods diet, you know that your energy level is already up to the brim. Naturally.

For those of you who may be brand-new to the world's best diet, or are about to begin, you're about to discover this for yourself.

A vegan diet, all by itself, keeps you bright-eyed and bushy-tailed.

Once you stop putting the flesh and blood and secretions of dead or captive animals into your system, you are no longer weighed down, slowed down by that stolen plunder. You are free to live a new life fueled by fresh nutrients, not the secondhand stuff, and you will find yourself invigorated in the most natural and healthiest possible way.

You won't need a lot of buzz drinks to force-start your body's engine.

You are already up for action. You have energy to spare. You are ready to rock and roll!

Whoa, simmer down, you.

Simmer down.

Happy Home Remedies That Make Use of Old Coffee Grounds

That's right, you can stop throwing them away and start putting them to use!

- Scrub your hands with wet coffee grounds to help remove strong odors like onion, garlic, and chile pepper.
- Remove stubborn grease and grime from dirty dishes by scouring with wet coffee grounds, using a scrubbing pad or a dishcloth.
- Hide scratches in dark wood furniture by dabbing them with wet coffee grounds, then wiping dry. Test first in an inconspicuous area to make sure the wood color is a suitable match.
- Deodorize your refrigerator by placing an uncovered bowl of dried coffee grounds on a shelf in a secure location where it won't be tipped over.
- Scatter old coffee grounds around plants and borders to help repel ants, snails, slugs, and other garden pests.

CHAPTER NINE

The World's Best Beverage

THERE IS ONE DRINK I ENJOY MORE THAN ANY OTHER, AND I NEVER CAN DRINK enough of it, I'm so fond of it.

You should drink more of it, too.

You really should. And I'm going to tell you how to do it.

First, I'll tell you what it is (though you have probably already guessed).

But wait. Let's recap a bit.

I've told you that I like strong drink and the occasional soft drink. I've sung the praises of coffee and tea in moderation. You also know that I love almost any flavor of unsweetened, caffeine-free herbal tea, served piping hot or ice cold. Naturally, I adore all fruit and vegetable juices, because I adore all fruits and vegetables.

Not one of these aforementioned drinks is my favorite, however. No, indeed. If I had to choose but one thing to drink for the rest of my life, it certainly would not be wine or beer or root beer or coffee or tea or juice.

No, it would be water—pure, clean water, the world's best beverage. That's my favorite, and I'm not just saying so because water is essential to life—though that is a very good reason.

In fact, anyone foolish enough to pick Coke, or carrot juice, or anything else but water as the sole beverage for the rest of their life would have a very short rest of their life, I'm sorry to say.

I also pick water as my favorite drink because I love the way it refreshes me and makes me feel good all over. I also love the taste of water, as long as it tastes like nothing. That's the perfect flavor for water. It should be clear and clean and fresh, like the air we want to breathe.

Just as we don't want a lot of difficult smells in our air, we also don't want a lot of puzzling flavors in our water.

Unfortunately, the municipal tap water that comes out of the faucets in our homes or the drinking fountains in town is sometimes flavored in ways that disappoint us, to say the least. It is still water, and unless there is something seriously amiss at the water treatment plant, it is avowedly safe and better than nothing.

But, it is not water at its best.

I used to make fun of bottled water when it started becoming so popular a few decades ago. Why were people paying boutique prices for the stuff that covers most of the Earth's surface free of charge?

But I swear, tap water has started tasting worse and worse as time goes by, at least to me, and now I'm grateful for the fact that there's a whole aisle at the grocery store that is stocked with bottled water of every shape and size and price.

Well, I'm mostly grateful, I should say.

It's a bit of a sore point for me personally, considering where I live. I can walk out into my front yard and see the famous arrowhead rock formation carved by nature into the foothills of the San Bernardino Mountains in Southern California. "The Arrowhead," as it is called, is California State Natural Landmark No. 977 and it is the namesake not only for Lake Arrowhead above it, on the mountaintop, but also of Arrowhead Springs below it, an artesian oasis where bottled Arrowhead Mountain Spring Water has been sourced since 1903.

I see the tanker trucks coming and going, filling up with perfect water that is transported all over the Western United States and enjoyed by millions of people.

Since I live downhill in the valley just below the fountainhead of this remarkable water, I figure my tap water should be awesome. Right?

Alas, the tap water is clear and bright only some of the time, while other times it comes out in various shades of gray, or even brown, or even red. And it ranges in taste from OK to terrible with flavor notes that can be described variously as metallic, tanky, rusty, swampy, and soapy.

I sigh, heavily, as I turn the tap on, then off. And later I grumble, a lot, as I pay good money for bottled Arrowhead Mountain Spring Water at the store. I wish I could just trudge up the hill a little ways, with a pail, and get the good stuff that comes out of the magic spigot there, within sight of my house. Unfortunately, it's a tightly guarded location.

Oh, well.

In spite of my grumbling, I do admit that I am willing to pay whatever it takes to have good water to drink.

It's vital. It's the world's best and most necessary beverage. And it's my favorite.

You see, I come from a long line of water drinkers.

You won't be surprised to hear that Seventh-day Adventists in general are big aquaphiles (yes, that's a word!). It started at the beginning, with Ellen G. White. You're not surprised to hear that, either, are you?

"Pure water is one of heaven's choicest blessings," my great-great-grandmother wrote in *The Ministry of Healing* (1905). "Its proper use promotes health. It is the beverage which God provides to quench the thirst of animals and man. It helps to supply the necessities of the system, and assists nature to resist disease."

Now, when I was growing up, the Weeks family refrigerator was stocked with very few things to drink. There was milk, which I always disliked. I would pour it sparingly on cereal, but I didn't care to drink it by the glass, ever. There often was a quart of buttermilk, too, in the family fridge, because my dad was fond of it. I have forgiven him for this. He was a good man. But honestly, buttermilk is the ghastliest last thing in the world I ever would pour down my own throat. In fact, I loudly hated it so much even in childhood that my parents learned to deploy it as a device of punishment. If I misbehaved in some extreme way, I was forced to drink a tall glass of buttermilk. It was like torture.

I also hated cottage cheese, another nasty lumpy dairy product, so my parents also implemented this as a deterrent weapon. A compulsory serving of cottage cheese was way more effective than a hard whipping in making me repent my sins.

I think we can glean two important truths from this whole business with the buttermilk and the cottage cheese.

First, my parents were sadistic monsters.

Ha! I am just joshing, of course. What I mean to say is that my parents were clever and ingenious tacticians in establishing discipline in their household.

Second, we also can surmise from this business with the buttermilk and the cottage cheese that I was greatly ahead of my time in perceiving the manifest dangers of consuming dairy products. Either that, or I was just lactose intolerant. We never will know, because I have shunned most dairy products by choice for most of my life, so their physical impact on me never has never been fully tested.

Anyway, let's get back to business here. We were talking about the beverage contents of my family fridge when I was growing up. Usually, in addition to milk and sometimes buttermilk (ick!), there was juice of some kind. Orange or apple or grape.

That's about it.

There never was soda pop, either the caffeinated kind because of the caffeine, or any other variety because of the sugar. We would have root beer floats as a special treat, now and then, but we would go out for those. There never was root beer in the house.

And, of course, there was no tea or coffee.

Sometimes I would complain, "There's nothing to drink!" as I opened, then closed the refrigerator door, dejectedly.

"Just drink water," Mom would say. She said it a million times.

And that's what I did. I just drank water. A million times.

We didn't splurge on bottled water in those days. We drank it out of the tap. Straight. We didn't even put ice in it. Or keep a pitcher of it in the fridge.

I guess Mom believed that good plain water was good enough.

She got it from her dad.

Herbert C. White, my grandfather, wrote more about water even than Ellen G. White, his grandmother, ever did. In his book *Nature's Seven Doctors* (1962), co-written with Dr. H. E. Kirschner and published under his own imprint, H. C. White Publications, water gets top billing.

It is one of the seven essential agents of health discussed in the book (along with sunshine, fresh air, good food, exercise, rest, and an active mind), but it gets four chapters of its own, more than any other.

Water has an "almost magic power" to promote health, prevent sickness, and reverse disease, my grandfather wrote. Many examples are offered of how water has been used throughout history to treat the body, both internally and externally.

Dr. Kirschner was personally acquainted with Dr. John Harvey Kellogg, who for decades was director of the Adventist-founded Battle Creek Sanitarium in Michigan. Hydrotherapy was high on the list of therapeutic services offered at the institution (not surprising, since Kellogg himself was author of a massive book titled *Rational Hydrotherapy*, published in 1918). Patients were treated with copious amounts of water both inside and outside their bodies. Cold baths, hot baths, sitz baths, cabinet baths, "fomentations" (hot and cold wet compresses), wet sheet wraps, water massages, and colonic irrigation and cleansing were among the extensive water applications available.

The sanitarium grew from little more than 100 patients during its first year of operation (1866) to more than 7,000 annually during its heyday in the early 1900s.

Indeed, "The San," as it was called, became famous and attracted a clientele that included such luminaries as President Warren G. Harding, President William Howard Taft, former first lady Mary Todd Lincoln, aviator Amelia Earhart, Ford Motor Company founder Henry Ford, J. C. Penney founder James Cash Penney, human rights activist Sojourner Truth, playwright George Bernard Shaw, actor and athlete

Johnny Weissmuller, and even C. W. Post, founder of Post Cereals, which competed with the cereal company founded by Kellogg and his brother W. K. Kellogg.

In fact, Dr. Kellogg would later accuse Post of stealing the recipe for Kellogg's Corn Flakes while he was a patient at Battle Creek. Post had crept into Kellogg's office and burglarized his safe, the good doctor claimed!

OK, that's enough about corn flakes. Let's get back to hydrotherapy. And when I say hydrotherapy, I don't mean sitz baths, though don't let me stop you if you enjoy those. But, no, I am talking about the health benefits of water taken in its simplest form. In a drinking glass.

Lots of drinking glasses. Every day.

We need it.

You see, humans are just big, complicated bags of water, so yes, water is very, very important. It's the main ingredient in our bodies and it accounts for about 60 percent of our body weight. It's what keeps every system in our bodies lubed and lively. It transports nutrients to the cells where they are needed and flushes toxins and wastes away from our vital organs.

And, mind you, we humans are not watertight. Not at all. We are big, leaky bags of water. We lose water when we breathe, when we talk, when we sneeze, when we sweat, and when we relieve our bladders and bowels. We are losing water all the time, so consequently we need to replenish water all the time. It's what makes us work.

The old adage, "Drink eight 8-ounce glasses of water a day," is a useful formula, and easy to remember, but it's important to remember that circumstances and individual needs do vary. If you are exercising and sweating on a hot or humid day, or if you're huffing and puffing at high altitude, or if you're pregnant or breastfeeding, or if you're sick and feverish and losing fluids due to vomiting or diarrhea, you obviously need extra water.

The "drink when you're thirsty" rule is a good one, but unfortunately there are millions of people who are so chronically dehydrated that they don't recognize thirst as soon as they should. Here's what the

Mayo Clinic Health Letter has to say on the subject: "Don't use thirst alone as a guide for when to drink. By the time you become thirsty, it's possible you may already be slightly dehydrated."

Fortunately, you don't have to worry about becoming parched, because you are going to hydrate properly. I'm going to show you how.

First, if you haven't started doing so already, consider eating the world's best diet, which is full of juicy fruits and vegetables like tomatoes and watermelon and grapes and cucumbers and carrots that are as much as 90 percent water. If you're eating right, you're getting up to one-quarter of your daily water needs from your food alone.

The rest is easy!

Now, I know, if you were to fill up eight separate tumblers with 8 ounces of water each, and line up those eight tumblers in a row, and look at those 64 ounces of water all at once, it would be a daunting sight.

So, don't do that.

Take it nice and slow. Drink a glass of water when you wake up each day. You can manage that, can't you? It's just one glass of water, and it's a great way to power up and get started.

It also will help you moderate the temptation to rely too much on coffee or tea in the morning. That's also a good thing.

If you feel like having an extra glass of water with or after breakfast, great, go ahead. If not, don't worry about it.

But remember to take a mid-morning break (you're OK with taking breaks, right?) and enjoy another glass of water while you do.

Later, when lunchtime rolls around, have a glass of water before you eat. It will get your juices going and start the process of filling your tummy even before you start adding calories. Have another glass of water while you eat. More swallows of water can mean fewer swallows of food you will need to satisfy your appetite. That's good!

And, besides, it's important to stay hydrated during that long middle of the day.

In fact, during your mid-afternoon break, refresh yourself with another glass of water. Keep those batteries topped up!

Later, when it's time for dinner, have a glass of water before you eat. It cleanses the palate and takes that first edge off your hunger. Calorie-free!

Feel free to have another glass or two of water during dinner. It's the world's best beverage, remember. A twist of fresh lemon or lime adds a nice touch and looks pretty in the glass.

Next, enjoy your evening. If you exercise, or work on projects, or do chores, or do anything that makes you thirsty, you know what to drink, right?

In fact, as part of any good exercise regimen, or any bout of physical labor or exertion, it's wise to drink water before, during, and after.

OK, finally, it's time for bed. A glass of water before retiring will help your body's engine hum while it idles. It will make your tummy feel good and help your muscles relax. You'll sleep better and dream better.

Before drifting off, think back on your day and tally up the glasses of water you enjoyed. Wow, you drank somewhere between eight and a dozen glasses of water!

That was easy, wasn't it?

Not only easy, but oh-so-refreshing, too.

Here's an extra tip I've learned as a lifelong connoisseur of the world's best beverage: Ice water may be a special treat but it's not the best choice for efficient hydration. If you drink your water cool, not cold, you'll drink more of it. Guaranteed.

Don't get me wrong. Ice water is fantastic for sipping. I love it. If I try to glug ice water, though, I get a bad case of brain freeze. I don't love that so much.

Happy Home Remedies for Brain Freeze

Yes, this is the perfect time to share my painstaking research on the subject of brain freeze, or "cold-stimulus headache," as it is known to science. The collision between icy foods or drinks and the warm interior of your mouth can surprise nerve endings near your brain, triggering a sharp pain reaction. Sometimes, inhaling frosty air or diving into extremely cold water can produce the same result.

A typical cold-stimulus headache is harmless and subsides on its own within seconds. But that is small comfort to anyone who is in the throes of one. Here are steps you can take to prevent or shorten such episodes:

- The sensitive area is where the roof of your mouth meets the back of your throat, so try to avoid shocking that area. Enjoy your frozen treat slowly and deliberately. Avoid gulping. Savor each bite, each sip, on the front of your tongue instead of the back. Use a spoon instead of a straw to enjoy slushy frozen drinks. A straw can act like a pressurized hose, delivering the stimulus straight to the target with intensified effect.
- If you feel a cold-stimulus headache coming on, act quickly to restore warmth to the afflicted area. Reach in and touch the spot with your thumb. Or use your tongue. Try to curl it so you can use its warmer underside to make contact.
- Another way to warm up the interior of your mouth is to pant like a dog into the cupped palm of your hand.

Admittedly, there's nothing dignified about panting like a dog, or sticking a thumb in your mouth like a baby, but hey, brain freeze makes us do crazy things!

CHAPTER TEN

The Smoking Gun

IF YOU ARE A USER OF TOBACCO, CONGRATULATIONS!

You have a big edge over other people.

Yes, those other people must take a number of steps, over time, to double or triple their odds of living a longer, healthier life.

You, on the other hand, can do it in a single day. Actually, you can do it in one short minute.

You can do it right now.

Quit smoking, or chewing, or sniffing, or sucking, or whatever it is you do with tobacco, and boom, just like that, in an instant, you almost certainly will have doubled or tripled, or maybe even quadrupled, your chances for an extended life, a better life, a happier life.

Congratulations!

I know, I know. Quitting is not easy. The nicotine in tobacco is one of the most insidious, most enslaving drugs there is, and once you become its bitch, it's hard to get your life back.

But you know it's possible to quit. Just look around you.

Seriously. Look around you. Doesn't it seem like almost everyone has quit?

That means you can do it, too.

In a few decades, we've gone from a society where practically everyone smoked to a society where practically nobody does, at least not in public.

Remember when people smoked in restaurants, in movie theaters, on airplanes and trains and buses, in stores, in offices, in meeting halls—in fact, in just about every possible public place?

Now, throughout America and many other nations, there is almost no public place, anywhere, in which smoking is permitted.

Smokers are now the outcast minority, forced to retreat to ever smaller, ever more remote places to stink up themselves in isolation where polite society doesn't have to see them or smell them.

If you use tobacco, I'm sorry I just called you an outcast. But I also am offering you encouragement and praise.

Millions have quit. So can you.

That's the encouragement.

And good for you, for even thinking about quitting.

That's the praise.

And I know you are thinking about quitting, because that's what all smokers are always doing. They are always thinking about quitting.

Right?

OK, there may be a few unrepentant sinners out there who are proud of smoking and have no wish or intention ever to quit, but I never have met one, or even heard of one, so they must be rare indeed.

No, most smokers want to quit. That's why there are so many smoking cessation products and programs out there. In fact, I'll bet the smoking cessation industry is making as much money, if not more, than the tobacco industry these days, at least in America.

I can make this chapter of my book a short one, I think, because I don't need to do any preaching. All smokers are converts already. They have heard the message and accepted the truth. They believe!

We all know the truth. We all have seen the postmortem photos of smoke-blackened lungs. We all have seen the commercials that show haggard addicts croaking their sorry testimonials as they light up another butt and stick it in their surgically cut throat holes.

We all have heard the dire statistics: One of three tobacco users will die from the poison they willingly take. The use of tobacco is the top preventable cause of death. Most smokers live ten to fifteen fewer years than nonsmokers do.

No, it's not necessary for me to make a case against the use of tobacco. That job has been done. My job, in this chapter, is to tell the story of how I started using tobacco and how I quit it. If it helps just one person, I will feel gratified.

Oh, screw that. I won't feel gratified unless I help at least a billion people quit!

So, here goes.

Remember my boyhood pal Jay? The one who went on those scavenger hunts with me on the side of the road when we were nine or ten? Well, we didn't just look for booze bottles with a little alcohol left in them. We also looked for cigarette butts with a bit of tobacco left.

We found lots. Some of them had a good fourth of their original contents still intact. A few had almost half. Occasionally we would hit the jackpot and find a cigarette that barely had been puffed.

I guess a few people were trying to quit even back then.

Anyway, we would collect these treasures and disappear into the woods along the road, where we would light up our butts with kitchen matches from home and smoke away.

Yes, we were the debonair pair, sitting on dirt and sticks under the trees, living the good life, holding our smokes at just the right angle, like we saw it done in all the magazine advertisements and on television. So what if our cigarettes had been lying on the ground, and maybe were weather-beaten and damp, and maybe were muddy and dirty, and certainly had been in other people's mouths?

We were men of the world. Jet-setters. Playboys. Have there ever been more sophisticated nine-year-olds, either before or since?

I'm just throwing out the question.

Also, I am supplying the answer. No, in fact, we were just rotten little punks.

One time, we really jacked the system. I brazenly walked into a small convenience market (after casing the joint, of course, to make sure there were no other customers) and laid cash money on the counter.

"My father sent me to buy cigarettes," I lied to the clerk.

"Why didn't he come himself?" the clerk asked.

"He's sick," I lied.

It worked. "What kind does he want?" the clerk asked.

"One carton of Kool Menthols for while he's sick, and a carton of his regular brand, Marlboros, for when he gets better."

"Has he bought cigarettes here before?"

"All the time."

The clerk rang up the purchase, bagged up the cigarettes for me, and sent me on my way.

Jay was hiding nearby. We danced in triumph, hugging and laughing.

When I recall this story today, and think of my innocent father, my sweet, pious, nonsmoking father, who at the time was head of public relations for the entire worldwide Adventist church, famous for its temperance message, and how I misrepresented him as the kind of sick smoker and irresponsible father who would send his little boy out to buy cigarettes for him, it makes me blush with shame.

It also makes me giggle a little bit.

Fortunately, most of these ill-gotten cigarettes were never used. Nine-year-olds don't have a lot of good hiding places for contraband items such as these, so we came up with what we thought was the ingenious idea of burying them in the woods.

I know, it was idiotic. We went from smoking secondhand cigarettes we picked up off the dirt to smoking new cigarettes we dug up from under the dirt. And each time we unearthed our stash, we found that our smokes were becoming damper, and soggier, and harder to light, and more unpleasant to smoke. Soon, we buried them one last time and left them that way.

Thus did the great majority of our Kools and Marlboros perish in the soil. Ashes to ashes, so to speak.

This childhood escapade with tobacco came to an end, as the one with alcohol had done, with no hard-core consequences, at least in the short term. It would be years before I fooled around with smoking again.

In fact, in my preteens I received a small award when I entered a piece of original artwork in a national temperance contest, sponsored by the church, and it won! My drawing was a variation on the old cigarettes-as-coffin-nails concept.

Hold on, this was a long time ago. Maybe I INVENTED the cigarettes-as-coffin-nails concept. Maybe I should have won a HUGE prize!

Curses!

Later, when I was in high school, the campus hellions (and I was one of them) would smoke to be cool on occasion, especially after we became old enough to have driver's licenses and cars of our own in which to cruise around. If we felt daring enough, we would even smoke in our cars as we drove through Loma Linda—being careful, of course, to crack open the windows in order to vent the telltale plumes of smoke.

Full stops at red lights or crosswalks presented a special challenge, requiring us to fan the smoke madly with our free hand in order to dissipate it manually. When there were four or five of us guys in a single car, and all of us were doing this simultaneously, it made for a lively scene!

Because the use of tobacco is just about the worst choice a person can make, health-wise, it's no surprise that it's just about the top taboo, health-wise, within the Seventh-day Adventist church.

If you are an Adventist and you are spotted enjoying a steak dinner at some restaurant somewhere, there will be no consequences for you, in terms of your good standing in the church. Perhaps a bit of kidding and winking.

"I hope that was a soy-based vegetarian steak I saw you eating the other night!"

If you are spotted enjoying a glass of wine with that steak, you probably will earn nothing more than a raised eyebrow. And more kidding, perhaps.

"I hope that was grape juice you were drinking with your vegetarian steak!"

But if you are spotted beating the weed in the parking lot outside the restaurant, you probably can expect an imminent pastoral visit, or some other form of concerned intervention.

"Tobacco is a poison of the most deceitful and malignant kind, having an exciting, then a paralyzing influence upon the nerves of the body," wrote Ellen G. White in a book of 1864 titled *Spiritual Gifts*. "It is all the more dangerous because its effects upon the system are so slow, and at first scarcely perceivable. Multitudes have fallen victims to its poisonous influence. They have surely murdered themselves by this slow poison."

She was years ahead of her time on this issue. The U.S. Surgeon General didn't come out against tobacco until the 1960s, a full century later. Cigarette ads in magazines of the 1960s still featured doctors in uniform extolling this or that brand as offering the finest, smoothest smoke.

I know, I know. It's too bad I didn't pay more attention to the prescient admonitions of my great-great-grandmother. I knew the truth about tobacco long before it became a mainstream public topic, and I should have known better than to even fool around with the stuff.

I guess I'm not the first person to foolishly ignore the wisdom of an elder, but ignoring the wisdom of this particular elder was especially foolish, I have to admit.

My relatively brief stint as a serious smoker didn't start until I began my newspaper career in San Bernardino.

Newsrooms of that era were notoriously thick with smoke. There was a constant haze of black and blue and gray. It was almost hard to see. Everyone smoked. The sportswriters smoked cigars. The arts writers smoked pipes. Everyone else smoked cigarettes. There were ashtrays piled high with butts on every desk, not to mention deep cigarette burns gouged into the edges of every desktop. Sudden wastebasket fires were common, started by the careless discarding of smoldering butts or still-glowing pipe cinders.

Maybe it was almost in self-defense that I started smoking. I knew there was no escaping the fact that I would be breathing smoke all day. I figured it might as well be the smoke out of my own mouth instead of somebody else's.

But after a number of years of this, when I realized I was smoking more cigarettes a day than I ever intended, and sometimes buying cigarettes by the carton instead of the pack (and, alas, no longer digging holes and burying those cartons in the woods), I finally decided that enough was enough. There was even a bit of a cancer scare to fortify my decision. A troublesome patch of irritated tissue in my throat required a biopsy. I made an out-loud promise to heaven above that if the lesion were found to be benign I would quit cigarettes forever.

It was. I did.

And I have kept my promise for thirty years.

Here's how I quit. I used the bait-and-switch method.

You see, I believe there are two factors that make the use of tobacco so addictive. There's the nicotine, of course, which is a powerful narcotic drug. That's obvious.

But there also is the oral factor, the pacifying pleasure that we humans enjoy when we have something in our mouths upon which to suck. It is a powerful dependency, especially for people like me who have never fully outgrown our infancy. We're just big babies cleverly disguised as adults.

Sometimes not so cleverly.

When I quit cigarettes, I knew the craving for nicotine would be a bear. But I knew I would be better able to handle that challenge if I could quell that other need, the oral need.

I started by sticking an unlit cigar in my mouth whenever necessary. It did the trick as far as keeping my mouth occupied, and the fact that it eventually became mushy and disgusting was an added bonus. It felt good each time I finally took the darn thing out of my mouth and tossed it.

Excellent teaching moments!

Later, when I realized I still was sticking nicotine in my mouth, albeit in smoke-free form, I ditched the unlit cigars. I decided to stop kidding myself. (And, by the way, people who now indulge in the fad of "vaping," which is a technically smoke-free activity that involves sucking and spewing the nicotine-enriched steam that comes out of battery-powered vaporizers known as e-cigarettes, may be kidding themselves in a similar way.)

I graduated to an old, unlit, empty tobacco pipe. Sure, my friends and co-workers made fun of me and my unloaded weapon, but I ignored them with a serene silence that spoke volumes. Make fun of this dormant volcano, if you dare, but beware, my friends, for a mighty outcome is assured!

After a few weeks, or maybe months, of this silly exercise, I down-sized to toothpicks. Plain old toothpicks. I walked around with a tooth-pick in my mouth for so long that people started calling me "Tex."

But guess what? It worked. It was pretty easy, eventually, to quit the toothpick habit and, by then, I had kicked the tobacco habit, too.

Hurray!

I still have smoking dreams, now and then, so I guess it's still on my mind—lo, these many years later—but I'm proud to say that when I am smoking in a dream, and I suddenly notice it, it causes me great distress. "Oh, no!" I say, in my dream. "When did I start this again?"

I am furious with myself. How stupid I am, I think. Then, I wake up. Whew!

If you're a smoker, and you think the bait-and-switch method might help you quit, I urge you to give it a try.

Remember, the key is to calm down that raging oral fixation of yours by putting things in your mouth that aren't on fire or full of poi-son. Try the unloaded pipe trick. Try toothpicks. Try sugar-free mints. Try chewing gum. Do whatever it takes. Anything, really.

Suck on your thumb, if that's what you have to do.

Even better, for those of you with romantic partners, see if they occasionally will let you suck on their thumbs.

Or whatever.

A Happy Home Remedy to Help You Quit Tobacco

Believe it or not, a little math exercise might be what it takes to help you beat the habit. Just run a few figures and you'll find that tobacco is laying waste to your billfold as well as your body.

Tobacco is overpriced as well as poisonous, and that should give you all the extra incentive you need. If you won't do it for the sake of your health, do it for the sake of your wealth!

Check the arithmetic. Let's say you smoke about a pack a day and you pay about five bucks for each pack. If you stop now, you'll save the following amounts of money:

$5 in one day
$35 in one week
$150 in one month
$912 in six months
$1,825 in one year
$18,250 in ten years
$36,500 in twenty years

Of course, if you're smoking more than a pack a day, or paying more than $5 for each pack, or if the price of cigarettes goes up, these figures escalate in a hurry.

The bigger the figures, the bigger the reasons to quit, my friend.

CHAPTER ELEVEN

Exercise Your Right! (And Your Left!)

I HAVE A COUPLE OF OLD EXERCISE MACHINES SITTING UNUSED IN THE GARAGE. And everyone I know has one or more old exercise machine gathering dust somewhere. Probably everyone they know can say the same thing. And everyone they know. And so on.

What does this mean?

If everyone, everywhere, possesses one (or more) old, unused exercise machine (or machines), there currently are more of these machines on Earth than there are humans. They outnumber us. If they ever stir to life and organize against us, they will overpower us. Why, oh why, did we not exercise them to death while we had the chance, instead of leaving them alone to plot and scheme?

OK, I know what you are thinking. I may be exaggerating the danger. Maybe our old exercise machines are not conspiring to enslave us—yet.

But isn't that what they want us to think?

One thing is certain. Whether or not they present any real threat, these monstrosities have already cost us a lot of money over the years, taken up a lot of our space, and done us precious little good.

About twenty years ago, I received some unexpected bonus pay, and I was feeling flush one night as I watched late-night television. There may have been a couple of glasses of wine involved as well. I saw a commercial for an exciting new exercise machine that promised a full-body workout in only four minutes per day, available only for a limited time at the low, low price of $700.

A FULL-BODY WORKOUT IN ONLY FOUR MINUTES PER DAY? AVAILABLE ONLY FOR A LIMITED TIME? AT THE LOW, LOW PRICE OF $700?

Obviously, I had to have one.

Let this be a lesson to everyone. Drinking and watching late-night television don't mix.

The machine had a fancy name, but I ended up calling it the Torturer. It was a more appropriate appellation.

When it arrived, in several large, heavy boxes, I assembled the parts and discovered that it was the size of a subcompact car. It had a seat and pedals and grips and a bewildering array of wheels and slides and pulleys and levers and other mechanical (and maniacal) appurtenances that I now remember only reluctantly, and with a shudder.

Taking a seat within the hostile confines of the Torturer, then using both legs and arms to set it into lurching motion, produced an experience that gave me a vivid idea of what it would feel like if I were trying to paddle a canoe forward on dry land.

I quickly was able to ascertain that the Torturer's guarantee of a full-body workout in only four minutes per day never, ever could be challenged, because there is no way that even Arnold Schwarzenegger in his prime could have kept that thing going for four whole minutes.

I couldn't manage it even for one minute.

Of course, I only tried it a few times. And then I denounced the Torturer and forsook it forever.

In hindsight, what's even more embarrassing than the fact that I wasted $700 on that beast is the fact that it's still in my garage today, taking up a subcompact car's worth of space and becoming more and more of an eyesore as it gathers additional draperies of dust and spiderwebs, having not been touched in two decades.

Believe me, if exercise machines do one day rise up against their careless masters, I know it's the Torturer that will be coming after me. I have seen it in my dreams.

Now, I know there are machines less scary than that one, and I know there must be a few people out there who bought exercise machines years or even decades ago and still are using them. Frankly, I've never heard of such people, but I'm sure they exist, and bless their hearts, I say.

And if there are people who are getting their money's worth out of health clubs and gym memberships, bless their hearts, too. And if there are people who are working out to videos each day in their homes or lying on the floor and doing stomach crunches or yoga poses or anything of that sort, in a disciplined way, every day, bless their hearts, too.

Keep up the good work.

Me, I don't have the discipline or the patience to exercise that way. Or the pain threshold.

I can't maintain my interest in those kinds of exercises. Or my discomfort tolerance level.

I need something a little more clever than that, a little more painless, a little more fun to do.

In short, I need something better.

And, with apologies to those few brave gym rats and exercise buffs out there, I claim that most of the world's normal people are like me, not them.

And bless our hearts, too!

So, here's my exciting news.

There's a form of exercise that gives the whole body a workout, is endlessly engaging and interesting, is practical and useful, and for most people it is easy and painless to do.

We already do it every day. It's an intrinsic part of our routine. We just need to do a little bit more of it, that's all.

It's walking.

That's right, walking, the world's best exercise. And we're going to see how simple it is to step it up a notch so that it does more than just get us here and there. It can take us to a whole new level of health and fitness!

Exercise is important. In the same way that we need to eat well to keep our bodies properly fueled, we need to exercise well to keep our bodies finely tuned and in proper running order. Here's a recent statement from the *WellBeing Newsletter* published by Loma Linda University Health, the umbrella organization that manages all of LLU's programs and services: "Routine exercise reduces the risk for chronic disease and disability and helps treat some chronic conditions for those who do develop them. Moderately fit men and women halve their risk for type 2 diabetes, high blood pressure, heart disease, obesity, and some cancers."

Long ago, humans didn't worry about fitness. They didn't have to sweat it. That's because they were already sweating for other reasons. They had to work every bone and muscle in their body every day just to exist. They hunted and gathered their own food. They built their own shelters. They made their own clothes. Whatever it was they needed or wanted, they had to grow it or find it or make it themselves. By hand.

We don't need to worry about that stuff. We have laborsaving devices and modern conveniences. We are plugged in and powered up. We have cars. We have computers. We have credit cards. We barely need to lift a finger to get whatever we want.

That's the trouble. We don't have to exercise, which means we definitely do have to worry about fitness. We do have to sweat it. We literally have to force ourselves to exercise, because we no longer do it naturally, the way our distant ancestors did.

Walking is something of a sweet exception, of course, because it is something we still naturally do, just as our distant ancestors did. We simply need to do more of it. We might never do as much of it as they did, but if we do enough, we can make a full-fledged exercise of it, and take new advantage of an old necessity.

Mind you, walking for exercise means more than an occasional stroll around the block. It means the kind of walking that boosts your heart rate and makes you pant a little bit. A little sweat is OK, too.

Walking for exercise is particularly good for you. It boosts your cardiovascular health, strengthens your bones, improves your balance and coordination, stimulates your metabolism, burns calories, and lifts your spirits.

It's a head-to-toe exercise that makes you stronger and healthier, both physically and mentally.

"I have two doctors—my left leg and my right," wrote the great British historian George Macaulay Trevelyan in a 1913 essay titled "Walking." "When my body and mind are out of gear, I know that I shall have only to call in my two doctors, and I shall be well again!"

Now, some people have mobility issues. They don't have the full use of their legs. But even they can take advantage of the basic concept here. I say to them, whatever you use to get around, use it harder, use it more cleverly. Put more of yourself into it. I've seen people in wheelchairs who are remarkably fit and robust. They really give their wheelchairs a workout, and their wheelchairs give them a workout in return.

If you ride a scooter, don't just sit in it. Work the parts of your body that work. Rock your midsection, twist your shoulders, wave your arms. Do the Locomotion!

The general idea here, for each one of us, is to maximize—in a healthy, strengthening way—the organic efforts we make to propel our bodies forward.

For most people, that organic activity is walking. Other than the wiggling and crawling that we do as babies, walking is our first form of exercise, and throughout our lives, it continues to be the best. The authors of the book *Nature's Seven Doctors*, Dr. H. E. Kirschner and my grandfather, Herbert C. White, enthuse at great length on the topic of walking in their chapters on exercise:

"Yes, my friends, whether you are sick or well, if your daily schedule does not include time out for walking, you are missing one of Mother Nature's most precious blessings. In choosing a spot for your daily walk, get out into the country—as far as you can get from the noise, dirt, and traffic of the city. And don't forget to throw off as many clothes as possible while you are enjoying this marvelous health restorer—WALKING."

Like grandfather like grandson, I guess, because, sure enough, I always have been an avid walker, though I may not be as eager as my grandfather to "throw off as many clothes as possible." In fact, I am trying very hard right now to avoid mentally picturing my grandfather with his clothes thrown off.

Also, I don't think of walking as an activity for which you take "time out." I don't think in terms of taking a single "daily walk." I take lots of walks every day. Dozens of them. The more the better. Short ones, long ones, medium ones.

Also, I don't need to "get out into the country" to take a walk (remember, I am not half-naked, for one thing). No, I enjoy a walk wherever and whenever it is possible.

But I will say this. I have been blessed to live for most of my life within hugging distance of the trees and trails of the San Bernardino Mountains. I've crisscrossed these peaks. I have walked all the way, on more than one occasion, to the summit of Mt. San Gorgonio, also called Greyback, which at an elevation of more than 11,500 feet is the tallest mountain in Southern California.

Now, mind you, this is official walking, complete with heavy-duty hiking boots, a rucksack, and a stick. And there is nothing more wonderful. But there also are other kinds of walking that aren't long adventures involving planning, preparation, and gear.

I often walk to the big supermarket that is a mile from my house, as long as the grocery list is short and there won't be too many items for me to schlep home. Round trip, that's a nice two-mile walk right there, and it's not a big official "daily walk." It's just a grocery trip. It's part of the routine.

I go for shorter walks, too. When I started working at the newspaper, it was located in an old historic building downtown that didn't have an elevator. Everyone had to climb a flight of stairs to get to the second-floor newsroom. For years I stumped up and down those stairs a dozen times a day, at least, which means many dozens of times a week and hundreds of times a month.

Years later we moved uptown to a brand-new building and, once again, the newsroom was on the second floor, but now there was an excellent elevator as well as a staircase. Most of my colleagues crowded into that elevator, but not me. I kept using the stairs, and I never tired of pointing out to the folks who took the elevator that I made it up faster than they did. Plus, I was getting good exercise. Yes, I'm sure they were very jealous (even if they didn't act like it).

I also get plenty of exercise on the home front. I love walking a mile or two or three around the neighborhood, making sure the houses are still standing in place and all is well. Often I will explore a little farther, or even a lot farther, and sometimes I will discover little side streets and back alleys I don't remember seeing before, if I ever did.

I don't just check out the houses and the yards and the cars and the cats and dogs and people. In fact, I usually gaze upward, above and beyond the rooflines, because there are mighty mountains everywhere to be seen. The San Bernardino Mountains loom in the north, the San Gabriel Mountains in the west, and the San Jacinto Mountains in the east.

Sometimes I look down, especially when I find a coin on the street. Usually it's just a penny but occasionally it's a nickel or dime, or even a quarter, and then I really get interested. My head stays down for the rest of that walk!

I keep these coins in a jar and count them up at the end of the year. The total is just a few bucks, usually, but I remember one year when it was more than $20! I guess there were a lot of people with holes in their pockets that year. Or maybe I was just walking more. Bless my heart!

I'm still taking those walks, and I'm still finding and saving those coins. I figure if I keep hard at it, I eventually may save up enough money to make up for that $700 I blew on the Torturer!

Honestly, I don't know how many thousands of miles I've walked in my life, but I've picked up a few tips along the way, which you might find useful if you'd like to do more walking yourself:

- Before beginning your trek, limber up with some simple stretching exercises. Do a dozen arm circles. Maybe a couple dozen. Do a dozen marching-style high steps. Maybe a couple dozen. Get loose, then get going!
- Wear appropriate shoes. Flip-flops or sandals? That's not enough. Hiking boots? That's too much, unless you are walking on a rutted, rocky wilderness trail. For ordinary walking, get yourself a lightweight, comfortable shoe that fits well. It should be flexible enough to twist in your hand, but sturdy enough to provide support for the long haul. If you have to cut short a walk because your shoes are hurting your feet, those aren't the right shoes.
- Taking the dog for a walk is fun, but it probably is better exercise for Bowser than it is for you. All that stopping, waiting, scolding, and supervising is cutting into your time. Go ahead and take Bowser for his walk. But then take one of your own, too.
- Don't just walk on level ground. Take on a few steep hills or streets. Going uphill exercises one set of muscles and going downhill exercises a whole different set. And remember, exercising your lower body in different ways is also exercising your upper body in different ways. You are turning yourself into a well-oiled machine, my friend!
- Don't text and walk. A study in Australia found that walkers thus distracted are more likely to slow down, stoop, swerve, and stumble. And look stupid, I might add.

Walking is great for brainstorming. I learned years ago that if I am puzzling over a problem or looking for fresh ideas on any subject, a good walk often will lead me to a solution. I was happy to learn recently that science has corroborated this phenomenon. A study based at Santa Clara University in California, reported in the *Journal of Experimental Psychology*, found that subjects in various controlled experiments were able to generate more and better creative ideas while walking than while sitting.

"Walkers had more thoughts and a higher density of creative thoughts than sitters," said Marily Oppezzo, a professor of psychology and the study's lead author.

Here's one last tip. Tracking devices, including old-school pedometers and more high-tech digital gadgets, can be a great encourager, or a great discourager. Find out for yourself whether or not you are able to form a productive relationship with one. A Stanford University study showed that walkers who tracked their steps increased their workout by about 25 percent over walkers who didn't keep track. But remember, the effort to achieve large numbers can be daunting, too.

The fabled 10,000 steps a day is something of a Holy Grail for serious walkers. It amounts to about five miles and, if you are wearing a tracking device, you can keep score. That can be a good thing or a bad thing.

Don't try to go from zero miles to five miles on your first day, for heaven's sake. Work yourself up to it. And don't fret if you aren't achieving the Holy Grail every day. Sheesh. Who does that?

In fact, skip those tracking devices if you feel they're putting too much pressure on you. Just use your watch and your own good sense. Walking at a good clip will yield one mile every twenty minutes, give or take, depending on the length of your stride and the steadiness of your gait. Walk thirty minutes and that's a mile and a half. Good for you. Walk an hour and that's three miles. Congratulations. Take it one step at a time. Walk an hour and forty minutes and that's five miles. That's 10,000 steps. That's the Holy Grail. Welcome to knighthood!

A Happy Home Remedy for Blisters

First, don't get blisters. Blisters are a bummer. Blisters are punishments, and walkers don't deserve punishments, they deserve rewards.

Experienced walkers don't get blisters. Their feet are well-conditioned and their shoes are well-chosen.

But let's say that you're new to the walking game, you do too much too soon, and you discover too late that your shoes definitely are not made for walking. Here's what to do:

Don't poke or pop the blister. This could complicate the recovery by causing infection or forcing the formation of a secondary blister, thus restarting and delaying the healing process. If the blister has popped on its own, gently clean the wound and apply a disinfectant.

Pain and minor inflammation can be treated by soaking the wound in cold green tea or gently applying apple cider vinegar, tea tree oil, or aloe vera gel.

To prevent additional abrasion, take a piece of thick adhesive moleskin, available at pharmacies and markets, and use scissors to cut a hole in the middle that matches the size of the blister. Apply the bandage strategically so that the hole is over the wound, leaving it uncovered and able to breathe, but surrounded by a wall of protection against additional abrasion.

Wait until your blister heals, then start walking again, preferably into a shoe store in search of good walking shoes that fit your feet comfortably.

CHAPTER TWELVE

Gardening— Reap 'Em and Eat

I RECENTLY BOUGHT A T-SHIRT THAT SAYS, "GARDENING IS CHEAPER THAN therapy and you get tomatoes."

Cute, huh? And it's so true.

It also could be worded like this, giving it a different spin: "Gardening is good exercise and you get tomatoes."

Yes, gardening is a productive activity on so many levels. It tones our bodies and tunes our minds. It grounds us. It helps connect us to our roots as hands-on players in nature's drama.

And we get tomatoes.

The fruits and vegetables we grow ourselves are material blessings. They make a tangible contribution to our diet. The world's best diet, remember?

Gardening can be a year-round activity almost anywhere in the world. Why stop for winter when there are whole "winter crops" that include both fruits (persimmons, pomegranates, pears, grapefruits, tangerines, and more) and vegetables (winter squash, yams and sweet potatoes, artichokes, cauliflower, broccoli, beets, leafy greens, and more)?

Even in the most weather-challenged parts of the world, gardeners can achieve great success with indoor container gardens, or window-box herb gardens, or yard or carport greenhouses—or all of the above. Check out the possibilities. Portable, walk-in greenhouses made of fabric and/or plastic can be found on the internet for less than $100. Also, do-it-yourself building plans for sturdier greenhouses are available online.

There's no excuse to not garden!

My grandfather, Herbert C. White, was a zealous tiller of the soil. That's no surprise, considering that for years he was the garden editor of *Let's Live* magazine, a popular national publication.

He was fond of citing the Bible story of Adam and Eve and emphasizing the fact that they were gardeners, happily tending field and flower in the Garden of Eden.

The anecdote is repeated in the book he co-wrote with Dr. H. E. Kirschner, *Nature's Seven Doctors* (1962): "You will recall that our first parents were privileged to LIVE in a garden . . . We should profit by their good example, and spend more of our leisure time in the garden! If we do, great will be our reward in increased health and longevity."

I remember very well the visits we made to Grandpa and Grandma White's house when I was little. Each time, Grandpa would take us out back to admire his huge compost pile of smoldering black soil, and he loved nothing more than to surprise everybody with the latest prodigious vegetable or fruit he had picked from his plants and trees.

To this day I keep a framed photograph on display in my kitchen that shows my grandfather and his twin brother Henry grinning like big-game hunters as they pose on either side of a gigantic squash that is half as tall as they are.

Of course, a squash of that proportion isn't even good to eat, usually. It's full of woody pulp and freakishly large seeds. But my grandfather liked to grow one of those monsters now and then just to show off.

Seriously. He did it for effect. He did it for bragging rights. He wanted everyone to see what his hot-shot super soil could do.

He lavished endless attention on every detail of proper cultivation and planting. He would always say, "It's better to plant a fifty-cent tree in a five-dollar hole than to plant a five-dollar tree in a fifty-cent hole."

Gardening was in his blood. His grandmother, Ellen G. White, was herself a tireless gardener. "Exercise in the open air should be prescribed as a life-giving necessity. And for such exercise there is nothing better than the cultivation of the soil," she wrote in *The Ministry of Healing* (1905).

There are stories in my family of her toiling by lamplight in the middle of the night to plant flowers or vegetables while temperatures were cool, especially if there was a chance of morning rain. She planted spectacularly successful fruit trees, grapevines, and tomato plants in a distinctive way that involved digging deep trenches and bedding them with alternate layers of rocks and compost. The method was divinely inspired, she said. It had been revealed in one of the visions she received during the "night season" of sleep, as she called it.

She certainly managed to impress more than a few experts with this technique. Here's her story of an encounter with a nurseryman in Australia, where she lived for several years while spreading the Adventist message on that continent:

"While we were in Australia, [a] man of whom we purchased our peach trees told me that he would be pleased to have me observe the way they were planted. I then asked him to let me show him how it had been represented in the night season that they should be planted. I ordered my hired man to dig a deep cavity in the ground, then put in rich dirt, then stones, then rich dirt. After this he put in layers of earth and dressing until the hole was filled. I told the nurseryman that I had planted in this way in the rocky soil of America. I invited him to visit me when these fruits should be ripe. He said to me, 'You need no lesson from me to teach you how to plant the trees.'

"Our crops were very successful. The peaches were the most beautiful in coloring, and the most delicious in flavor of any that I had tasted" (from a letter of 1907, collected in *Selected Messages Book Three*, published posthumously in 1980).

Ellen G. White never hesitated to preach what she practiced as an active gardener. To her, gardening was much more than simply growing food to eat. She believed that gardening is wonderful therapy, with benefits for body, mind, and spirit. "Let men and women work in field and orchard and garden," she wrote. "Out-of-door life is a means of gaining health and happiness" (*Medical Ministry*, a collection of writings published posthumously in 1932).

As it happens, the gardening gene in my family has traveled all the way down to me. Like my great-great-grandmother, and like my grandfather, I love to go outside and dig in the dirt. It gives me a workout. It makes me feel happy.

And I get tomatoes!

Boy, do I get tomatoes. In fact, I'll make a little confession. I call myself a gardener, but unlike other gardeners who grow lots of different things, I only grow one thing. I'm a specialist.

I only grow tomatoes.

Mind you, I love all fruits and vegetables, but I'm not tempted to grow most of them. The way I see it, they are plentiful in the markets, they're affordable, and they taste just as good as the ones I could grow in my yard. So, why bother?

Tomatoes, however, are different.

The modern commercial tomato has been ruined by corporate agribusiness. It has been bred for mass production, uniform appearance, rock-hard transportability, and ageless shelf life—and flavor has been sacrificed in the process. It's a sad story told eloquently in the book *Tomatoland: How Modern Industrial Agriculture Destroyed Our Most Alluring Fruit* by Barry Estabrook (Andrews McMeel Publishing, 2011).

Today's factory-farmed tomatoes have been stripped of nutrition, too. Estabrook cites U.S. Department of Agriculture data that indicates the commercial tomatoes of today contain 30 percent less vitamin C, 30 percent less thiamin, almost 20 percent less niacin, and more than 60 percent less calcium than the tomatoes of the 1960s.

The sorry fact is that most of today's supermarket tomatoes don't deliver the goodness they once did. They don't nourish like they did. They don't smell like they did. They don't taste like they did. In fact, they don't even taste like tomatoes anymore.

They don't taste like anything at all.

Homegrown garden tomatoes, on the other hand, still taste heavenly. They taste like tomatoes are supposed to taste.

That's why I'm a tomato gardener.

I plant tomatoes all over the backyard, and I plant early in the season and late in the season so I can be inundated by tomatoes all summer long. I love to make salsa—tubs of the stuff—and then jar it up and store it in the cupboard. It's a great way to keep enjoying the tomato garden all year, even after the tomato garden is gone.

In a minute I'm going to share with you my recipe for John's Famous All-Red Salsa. Yes, I'm exaggerating when I call it famous, but I'll tell you what. I once wrote about it in a newspaper column and it started a little buzz on the internet. I started receiving recipe requests from all over the United States. Also, the recipe is included in a book—*City of San Bernardino Bicentennial Cookbook*, published in 2010. I guess that means it's a little bit famous, right?

(Oh, by the way, there also are plenty of other tomato-rich recipes, like Tomato Toast Tapas, and Layered Eggplant, Zucchini, and Tomato Casserole, coming up in chapter twenty-one of this book. The salsa recipe in this chapter is just a little appetizer!)

For years, in my garden, I planted only the popular tomato varieties that you find at all the garden centers and nurseries. I've had lots of luck with the Ace and Celebrity varieties, for example. Early Girls are pretty amazing, too. More recently, I've tried growing the more old-fashioned heirloom varieties. I found my inspiration for this at the spectacular Kendall-Jackson Heirloom Tomato Festival, held each September at the Kendall-Jackson Wine Estate and Gardens in Fulton near Santa Rosa, located in California's Sonoma County, just north of San Francisco.

It's a seven- or eight-hour drive for me, but I've made the pilgrimage every year for almost ten years because it's so awesome. There's a huge tomato-tasting tent, manned by an army of volunteers with slicing knives, where you can sample about 300 varieties of heirloom tomatoes of all shapes, sizes, and colors. There are bulging Oxhearts, striped Green Zebras, knobby Japanese Black Trifeles, and ready-to-burst

Brandywines. There are tomatoes that are corrugated like pumpkins, or elongated like cucumbers. There are tomatoes that are orange, purple, pink, or multicolored. There are tomatoes as big as melons and as tiny as peas.

Elsewhere on the festival grounds, you can sample delicious tomato appetizers paired with Kendall-Jackson wines. And around the perimeter of the festival grounds, there are booths where some of the Bay Area's finest restaurants offer tomato-inspired food samples.

It's a tomato orgy! (More info: http://www.kj.com/events/tomato-festival.)

As I say, I've been inspired to try planting heirloom varieties in my own tomato garden. They are fussier than the varieties I've planted in the past. They take a little more time and attention. I plant them, water them, fertilize them, prune them, babysit them with special care.

But that's OK. It's good exercise. It's good therapy.

And, I get tomatoes!

JOHN'S FAMOUS ALL-RED SALSA

About 6 cups

This salsa is made entirely of red or orange ingredients, so it's very bright and colorful. It's also very delicious. Of course, I use my own homegrown garden tomatoes, but any good red flavorful tomatoes will work.

> 10–12 medium to large red tomatoes, peeled and chopped
> 2 small red onions, chopped
> 1 large red bell pepper, cored and chopped
> 2–6 fresh habanero peppers, cored and minced (the more you use, the crazy-hotter it gets!)
> Salt to taste
> Sugar to taste (optional)
> 1–2 teaspoons olive oil (optional)

1. To peel the tomatoes, slit their skins in two or three places, and then drop into boiling water for about 30 seconds, until the skins start to blister. Remove the tomatoes with a slotted spoon and plunge into cold water to cool. The skins should slip off easily.
2. Combine and mix all the ingredients. Drain excess juice if thicker salsa is desired. Enjoy.

NOTE: The bell pepper and habanero peppers can be peeled, too, by fire-roasting them whole until blackened on a stove top or grill, plunging into cold water, then rubbing off most of the blistered skin. To core peppers, slice open and scrape out and discard the seeds and membranes. Use only the outer flesh of the peppers.

Happy Home Remedies Starring the Tomato

You already know that tomatoes are good for your insides. They're loaded with health-sustaining vitamins and minerals, plus disease-fighting antioxidants, beta-carotenoids, and amino acids. But did you know that tomatoes are good for your outsides, too?

Beautiful skin: Apply fresh tomato juice or rub fresh tomato slices onto skin to cleanse, remove dead skin cells, tighten pores, smooth wrinkles, brighten skin color, even treat acne and soothe sunburn.

Beautiful hair: Before showering, apply fresh tomato juice or tomato pulp to hair and massage into scalp. The longer you leave it in, up to a half hour, the better the results. This vitamin-packed, collagen-rich tomato treatment cleanses and conditions hair, removes odors, restores color and shine, replenishes moisture, treats dandruff and itchy scalp, and even guards against hair loss.

CHAPTER THIRTEEN

Sex—Long May It Wave!

OH, AND HERE'S ONE MORE EXERCISE THAT HAS PROVEN TO BE QUITE POPULAR. And effective.

Sex.

Sex burns about 100 calories during the course of an average half-hour session. That's 200 calories per hour, about the same as volleyball, ballroom dancing, or brisk walking, according to the Mayo Clinic.

That's good. And, of course, if you're having sex that is more robust than average, you are burning even more calories. And if you're going at it for more than an hour, well, hello, you really are making those calories disappear.

You also are making the rest of us extremely jealous.

Sex not only burns calories. It's also good for the cardiovascular system. And the immune system. It lowers stress. And it promotes sound sleep. These are wonderful health benefits.

As most of you probably know, sex also has another purpose. It is necessary for the perpetuation of the species. And, truly, it's the cleverest device in all of nature that the activity by which we produce offspring is also the activity by which we derive the most intense physical pleasure. Nature positively drives us to reproduce ourselves.

Sex is so much fun that we enjoy it even when procreation is not our goal. That's another major favor for which we have nature to thank.

Even for those who aren't actively trying to have a baby, and in fact even for those who absolutely do not want to have a baby, and in fact even for those who could not possibly have a baby even if they wanted one, sex is still fun. And good exercise.

Too old to make babies? No problem. Sex is still fun. And good exercise.

Infertile? Not an issue. Sex is still fun. And good exercise.

You may not be qualified technically to beget babies, but you still are qualified to derive all the pleasures, all the comforts, all the health benefits of sex—as long as you practice sex safely and responsibly, of course.

Sex is powerful. It is not only what makes the world go round, but it's also what got the whole thing spinning in the first place.

Whichever story of the origin of human life on this planet you may prefer, you must admit that it's a sex story from the get-go. Whether it was a matter of creation or evolution, somebody or something, somewhere, a long time ago, was having fun, fun, fun—and thus was life begun!

The Bible story, by the way, is especially sexy and, whether you read it as allegory or literal truth, you can't fail to notice that there's a short sex scene almost at the very beginning!

That's right, the second chapter of Genesis starts out with God taking a breather after His creation of the world, and feeling pretty good about things. But then He has an afterthought. Something's not quite right, He thinks. He has created a human being to live in the new world, but maybe there should be more than one. Hmmm. Maybe it should take two to tango in the Garden of Eden.

"The Lord God said, 'It is not good for the man to be alone. I will make a helper suitable for him'" (Genesis 2:18, New International Version).

So God creates a woman, Eve, to go with the man, Adam. And things immediately get interesting. There is full frontal nudity and everything!

"So the Lord God caused the man to fall into a deep sleep; and while he was sleeping, He took one of man's ribs and then closed up the place with flesh.

"Then the Lord God made a woman from the rib He had taken out of the man, and He brought her to the man.

"The man said, 'This is now bone of my bones and flesh of my flesh; she shall be called woman, for she was taken out of man.'

"That is why a man leaves his father and mother and is united to his wife, and they become one flesh.

"Adam and his wife were both naked, and they felt no shame" (Genesis 2:21–25, New International Version).

Like I said, it's a short scene. Way too short, in my opinion. I can't resist using my imagination to add details. To flesh it out, as it were.

Even Darwinians can enjoy the following exercise, I think. If you don't care to think literally of Adam and Eve as freshly created, fully formed human beings, just think of them metaphorically as whatever evolving primordial creatures you choose. Think of them as two tadpoles, if you like, or two salamanders, or two monkeys. Comfortable now? OK, let's rejoin the action in our "Newly Expanded Story of Adam and Eve, with Additional Mature Content Now Included, for Educational Purposes Only, to Better Illustrate and Elucidate the Importance of Sex in Explaining the Origin of Life on Our Planet":

Adam has seen much during the past few days, and it all is new to him, so he is neither startled nor afraid when he first sees Eve. Rather, he is enchanted to meet for the first time another creature so similar to himself, and yet also different.

Neither is Eve startled or afraid. Indeed, she is calmed and comforted to see a kindred form. He is like her in so many ways, but unlike her, too.

For some time they stand at a short distance from one another, gazing with curiosity and admiration at each other's naked bodies. There is no shame or embarrassment, just as there is no fear. Shame and embarrassment, like fear, are felt only by those whose hearts and minds have been tainted by Satan's sting, and Satan has not yet made an appearance in this story.

Adam and Eve say no words to each other, not yet, but they smile at each other. It gives them pleasure to do that. Smiling feels good.

Eve is the first to take several steps forward. She laughs, and the sound is beautiful to Adam's ear.

Adam now steps closer, too. He greets her. She loves the strong, deep sound of his voice.

When they are standing within reach of each other, Eve raises her hand and, without hesitation, places it on Adam's face. She touches his lips and is excited to see how it makes him smile even more happily. She feels his nose and chin, so much more prominent than hers. She traces with her fingertips the contour of his throat and lightly rubs the bump in the middle of it. She does not have a bump in her throat like that.

Next she explores his shoulders, so much broader than hers, and his chest, much flatter and more muscular than hers. She feels his nipples, smaller and harder than hers.

She slides her hands down and caresses his hips, so slender. She reaches behind and feels his buttocks, so small and compact compared to her own.

Finally, she examines the thing that has intrigued her the most, the one thing on Adam's body that bears no resemblance to anything on her own, the one limb that dangles between the two larger limbs that are his legs.

She reaches there and ruffles with her fingers the hair that sprouts above it, then she takes it in her hand and probes it, gently. She is amazed to feel it harden in her hand and grow larger.

Adam is amazed, too. He puts his hands on Eve's shoulders. He feels their roundness, so unlike the squareness of his own. He reaches up and touches her mouth, her lips so much fuller than his.

She kisses his fingertips, then impulsively leans toward him and they kiss on the mouth, not knowing why, but knowing that it is good.

Adam takes Eve's breasts in both hands and feels the weight of them, the heft of them. He caresses her pink nipples, large and soft, although they do grow harder as he touches them.

His hands stray to her hips and buttocks, and he feels how round, how voluptuous they are.

Next he reaches with one hand and touches the place between her legs, the mysterious place where there is no extra limb like the one he has on his own body. It's one of the first things he noticed about her and he is exceedingly curious.

His fingers explore the soft furrowed skin there and they find a moist crevice. Eve closes her eyes and murmurs with pleasure.

Adam's fingers glide easily now in that place and suddenly one finger sinks more deeply into an opening, and slides in.

They both exclaim. Adam's extra limb, still in Eve's hand, has grown to many times its original size. It is lifting upward at a sharp angle, and throbbing.

Desire consumes them. An idea occurs to both of them simultaneously. They realize that Adam's manhood and Eve's womanhood are interlocking parts that can be joined in a way that will please them both.

Spotting a flowery lawn in the shade of a nearby tree, they hurry there to put into practice the idea they have conceived.

And thus, dear reader, has so much been conceived ever since.

OK, OK, that's enough of this.

Whew! Somebody open a window! These Bible stories are HOT!

And, by the way, this is how any two creatures should love one another properly. They should treat each encounter as if it were the first. They should approach each other with interest, regard each other with admiration, touch each other with fascination, caress each other with eagerness, and enjoy each other with rapture and awe.

Again, while we don't need to agree on which origin story to believe, I think we must agree that nothing has changed in this matter since life on our planet began, however it began. Living creatures are hardwired with an essential interest in sex.

It's a curiosity, it's an itch, it's an unavoidable urge that dates back to the beginning of life in general, and to the beginning of each one of our lives in particular.

Sex is natural. And it's so easy to do it when we're young. (Too easy, perhaps.) We don't overthink it. We don't worry about the mechanics of it. We just do it. Boom.

Then we get older and we start sweating the details. We start over-analyzing. Maybe we're too old. Maybe we're too wrinkled and ugly. Maybe we're too dry. Maybe it will hurt. Maybe we don't have the energy. Maybe we can't get it up.

We get stupid about sex.

Sure, young people are stupid about sex, too, but it's a different kind of stupid.

Young people worry too little about sex and its consequences. Older people worry too much.

Here's my solution, and if I had a megaphone I would use it now:

Hey, young people, ponder sex a little more before you do it.

Older people, ponder less!

I've been fortunate enough to run into a number of older individu-als who have figured it out. And by "run into," you know what I mean.

I've had some wonderful long-term partners, as well as some won-derful short-term partners in the interims, and I'm happy to report that something remarkable happens for anyone of any age who is able to turn off the drama, tune out the performance anxiety, and let things happen.

Honestly, it wasn't until I had achieved middle age that I started to hear things like, "This is the best sex I've ever had," or, "Now I under-stand the big deal with satin sheets."

Believe me, I am no stud gun. I am just an average batter on this field of play, so to speak, so I never for a second have been tempted to regard statements such as these to be personal compliments directed at me.

No way.

Instead, these were the statements of people who have discovered, for themselves, a fundamental truth.

Sex can get better as we age.

Not worse. Better.

Young people are amateurs when it comes to sex. There's no artistry in the way they do it. It's just load-and-shoot, rooty-toot-toot! They aren't inventive at all. Maybe it's because they don't need to be.

As we get older, we want to be more cunning, more ingenious, more experimental because, well, we may need to be.

And there's no reason why we can't be.

We no longer need to worry about buzz-kill details such as menstrual cycles, birth control pills, intrauterine devices, or whatever. We can be headstrong and fearless. We can discover what the newbies, the amateurs, won't discover for years, if they ever do.

There are many sex organs and erogenous zones, not just the few we read about all the time. Our largest organ of all is our skin, which means we literally are encased from top to bottom and front to back with an impressively large sex organ that tingles at all times with millions of expectant nerve endings. Plus, there are the many digits, appendages, protuberances, orifices, apertures, crevices, and creases that can be found on our bodies, and they all can be brought into play. Tenderly. And lovingly.

I have many, many sex organs and erogenous zones on my body. And you have many, many of them on yours. If you can't think what they are, you need to count again.

Count your fingers, your toes, your knees, the back of your knees, your elbows, the back of your elbows, your shoulders, your hips, your thighs, your earlobes, your eyelashes, your tongue, your mouth, other openings here and there. Soft openings. Deep openings. All these places and things have nerve endings and they all can be thrilled. Tenderly. And lovingly.

I admit, I was a little bemused, even skeptical, perhaps, when I heard middle-aged ladies talk about having the best sex of their lives.

Sure, I took their word for it, but I didn't fully appreciate what they meant.

Then, something happened to me. As a middle-aged man I had a sexual experience for which nothing in the past had prepared me. It was beyond sexual, really. It was mind-altering. It was life changing.

It hit me midway through the act of doing it, though I'm just guessing about the timing, because what happened beforehand seemed to take place in normal time and what happened during it and what happened afterward were beyond timekeeping.

I no longer was in a room. I had left my body and I was a spirit form, flying above the world. I was glowing and full of light. Sparks flew out of me and trailed behind me like the tail of a comet. I was pure energy. Far below me I saw oceans, mighty mountains, dark forests, then a vast plain. I saw animals having sex on the savannah. I saw giraffes and lions and wild boars. I saw two zebras having sex. I loved the way their stripes rippled as they moved. I flew to them.

I became a zebra. First I was one of the zebras having sex. Then I became the other zebra having sex. Then I was both zebras having sex together.

I smelled the wet grass. I felt the hot sun on my back. The whole world stopped and there was just me, both of me, on the ground, with the blue sky above me. I was the only thing moving. I was the two zebras, moving, moving, our stripes rippling.

My real body, back in real time, in the real room, did have an orgasm during this real sexual experience. But it was almost unwanted. In fact, I tried to delay it. Or cancel it. It was a distraction to the greater thing that was going on. I knew that the orgasm would bring the experience, the vision, whatever it was, to an end.

And it did. But, thankfully, the aftermath lasted a long time. I was shivering in the bed, the real bed, in the real room, and I was shaking all over and moving my legs like a bicyclist does. And I was laughing. And crying. I was so happy. I was laughing and crying. Tears of joy.

Days later, long after I had returned to Earth and no longer was a rutting pair of zebras, I did some poking around—I mean, I did some investigating—to see if experiences such as mine had been reported by others.

To my surprise, I learned that my experience is not that rare, especially among middle-aged and even elderly people, and that there is quite a bit of research and literature on the subject. I can recommend one book in particular that I have read with great interest. It's called *Transcendent Sex: When Lovemaking Opens the Veil* (Gallery Books, 2004) by developmental psychologist Jenny Wade.

"The fact is, sex—all by itself—can trigger states identical to those attained by spiritual adepts of all traditions," she writes, "the animal possession and otherworldly travels of shamans, the bodily fireworks of kundalini yoga, the past-life revelations of reincarnation religions, the Void of Buddhism, and the 'unio mystica' described by Western saints."

The research of Wade (check out transcendentsex.org) and other investigators in this field indicates that mystical sex experiences occur in random fashion and in endless variety. They cannot be predicted or prompted. They are not an achievement, but more like a gift bestowed on those who receive them.

Of course, you have to play in order to win. There is no way to have transcendent sex without having sex!

And, while a high percentage of those who report such experiences are of mature age, these experiences can happen to young people, too.

In fact, they can happen to anyone, the researchers say. It makes no difference whether you're good in bed or lousy in bed, or whether you're male or female, straight or gay, religious or nonreligious, smart or dumb, strong or weak, even healthy or nonhealthy.

But, wait a minute. Even if health seems to be a nonfactor in the specific matter of so-called transcendent sex, it definitely is a factor in the matter of sex in general. And I want to take the opportunity here to work in one more plug for the world's best diet. (When I say "one more," I don't mean it will be the last!)

People who eat a plant-based whole foods diet are healthier than other people. And, generally speaking, healthier people make better lovers.

While I apparently do condone mingling intimately with mystical zebras during the course of a transcendent experience (honestly, I don't know what came over me that night . . . maybe I had been watching too many Animal Planet shows on TV), I never would think of putting carcass meat from a real zebra in my stomach.

It only makes sense that we are better able to be sexually alive if we are alive in every way, and we cannot be alive in every way if we feed on the dead.

This not only makes sense but it's also a proven scientific fact. It takes a healthy cardiovascular system to power the blood flow that engorges the male penis and the female clitoris. When everything works properly, magic happens. A damaged cardiovascular system, clogged by animal fat and cholesterol, is a poor performer, in more ways than one.

"Erectile dysfunction is actually the first clinical indicator of generalized cardiovascular disease. It's the canary in the coal mine," says Dr. Terry Mason, public health commissioner of Chicago, who appears in the documentary *Forks Over Knives*, as well as in a follow-up online film produced by the *Forks Over Knives* team that specifically addresses the link between diet and sexual health.

That short film, titled *Raise the Flag with a Vegan Diet* and viewable at forksoverknives.com, youtube.com, and many other websites, makes clear that the diet choices we make, on our own, are far more effective in improving our sexual function than the drugs prescribed by our doctors and dispensed by our pharmacies.

It's a power we have at any age. "I think connubial bliss up until one is eighty-five or ninety or one hundred should be, and ought to be, under our own locus of control," says Dr. Caldwell Esselstyn, another *Forks Over Knives* hero in the video.

Whether man or woman, we can "raise the flag" of our libido and sexual function by choosing a plant-based whole foods diet that charges up our life force to the max. Better health means better sex.

Not just better.

Biblical!

Happy Home Remedies for Sexual Dysfunction

Ginkgo biloba can improve blood flow everywhere in the body. That's right, everywhere, including the sex organs of both men and women. The herbal medicine has been used for centuries, not only as an aid to circulation but also as a treatment for anxiety and memory loss. The herb is an extract from the leaves of the ginkgo biloba tree, the world's most ancient, found in the wild only in China but now cultivated around the world. It is widely available in pill, powder, and liquid form at health food stores, pharmacies, large markets, and online.

Many other natural medicines with long histories of use in treating impotence and loss of libido are similarly available, including ginseng, evening primrose oil, flaxseed oil, L-arginine, and pomegranate. All have antioxidant properties that boost blood flow to small blood vessels.

Pomegranate, of course, is also available as a juice, which can be drunk daily for heart and blood health.

CHAPTER FOURTEEN

Sleep Well

I KNOW THAT ONE OF THE EARLIER CHAPTERS OF THIS BOOK IS TITLED "CHEATing in Moderation," but I don't believe in cheating one bit when it comes to sleep. If I don't get seven or eight hours of sleep each night, I get cranky and stupid.

Or crankier and stupider, depending on your opinion of me.

I run into lots of other cranky and stupid people all day, every day, and I figure I know what's wrong with them. They aren't getting enough sack time.

I actually feel ill when I'm running short on sleep, which is why I don't let it happen. I want a full night's worth. Even five or six hours aren't enough. I'm not satisfied. And I sure don't kiss the missing hours good-bye. No, I make them up the very next night, or at least as soon as possible. I'll take naps during the day if it's necessary. Whatever is required. I keep my sleep debt paid!

I believe that the quality of our sleep is as important to our good health as the quality of our diet. And there's science to back me up.

"Untreated sleep disorder symptoms may cause significant health problems and reduce quality of life," states a report by the Sleep Disorders Center at Loma Linda University Medical Center. Those problems include obesity, diabetes, heart disease, stroke, erectile dysfunction, dementia, depression and other mood disorders, and temporary impairment of everyday cognitive and physical functioning. Since 1982, the sleep center at LLUMC has offered diagnosis and treatment of afflictions that include insomnia, sleep apnea, snoring, narcolepsy, sleepwalking, nightmares, and restless leg syndrome. (More info: lomalindasleep.org.)

An estimated 40 million Americans suffer from chronic insomnia and/or other sleep complaints. Both adults and children are among the afflicted.

Sleep is a mysterious thing. I'm not exactly sure why we need as much of it as we do. I mean, eight hours is a third of the day. That's a lot of downtime. If we bought a car or a computer or any other device that shut down that often, we would consider it defective. We would turn it in for a refund.

Unfortunately, we can't turn ourselves in for a refund. We have to make the best of what we've got.

I suspect our sleep cycle derives from the fact that we live on a planet where it's dark roughly half the time. Our ancestors got used to going to bed when the sun went down, and we inherited the habit. Remember, our forebears didn't have fancy electric lights, like we do, so they had little choice. When it got dark, the day was done. Yes, there are a few things that are fun to do by candlelight, but it's a short list.

Just as we have inherited the habit of winding down after the sun sets, we also take after our ancestors in feeling compelled to rise with the sun. Well, most people do, anyway. I have to admit, it's a compulsion I personally do not share.

I understand that every second of daylight was important to the hunters and gatherers of long ago. They needed to work from dawn to dusk to get their job of survival done. What I don't understand is why we continue to force ourselves to get up every day while it's still dark and race off to work as the sun comes up. Despite our many advances, we seem to have the time management skills of cave people.

I am proud to say that I have not used an alarm clock in decades. They were a necessary evil when I was young. That school bell rings early! But I vowed that after high school, after college, after graduate school, when I finally was all grown up and could call my own shots, I never would use one again.

I try to keep most of my vows, and I certainly have kept that one.

Fortunately, I sought a career in the newspaper business, at a time when newspapers were in their heyday, with morning and afternoon editions and round-the-clock shifts. I was hired as a "night-side" reporter, working 4 P.M. to midnight, and a pattern was set. In later years, as newspapers struggled to survive in a new media landscape transformed by computers, and afternoon editions were discarded and morning editions were subjected to earlier and earlier deadlines, I had to accept modifications to my schedule. But I resisted every step of the way and did my best, always, to work as late a shift as possible. Once a night-sider, always a night-sider.

As a result, I have always been a very well-rested human being.

I loved the 4 P.M. to midnight shift. It seemed to me, then and now, like the perfect schedule, and I wondered why the whole world wasn't on it. I could stay up as late as I wanted, after work, and howl at the moon until all hours. Most of my friends were night owls, too, so there was always plenty to do. When I did go to bed, whether it was 2 A.M., or 3 or 4 A.M., or even sunrise, I fell asleep with a smile on my face because I knew I could sleep in as long as I wanted. No alarm clock was needed. And then, after I awoke, of my own volition and fully refreshed, there usually was plenty of time to get stuff done before I had to report for work. I could run errands, shop for groceries, do a little yard work or attend to other chores, or heck, just go for a long walk or relax and catch up on my reading. I didn't have to be at work until 4:00 in the afternoon, after all!

Because my schedule was so off-kilter from that of most other people, I never experienced traffic jams or crowded stores. It's like I had the world to myself. It was grand!

Now, I understand that everyone can't suddenly go on the night shift, just like that, and throw away their alarm clocks forever. But I also know that it is very much possible for each person to take steps to avoid alarm clocks, whether it is tweaking their schedule in favor of sleep, or going to bed earlier, or falling asleep more quickly, or sleeping more soundly, or preferably all of the above.

Alarm clocks are evil. If you are using one regularly to force yourself awake, against your will, you are not getting enough sleep. There's no other way to look at it.

What's worse, if you are one of the millions of people who are taking sleeping pills or other drugs to force yourself to sleep in the first place, and then relying on that alarm clock, a mechanical device that functions much like a drug, to force yourself awake from sleep, and then using coffee or other drugs to force yourself to perform despite your exhausted condition, then you are existing in a drug-addled zombie state that is not conducive to a long, healthy life—or anything else, for that matter.

Sufficient rest is one of *Nature's Seven Doctors* that is featured in the 1962 book of that title co-authored by my grandfather, Herbert C. White.

"Sleep is the Great Restorer," he writes. "Time spent in sound, refreshing sleep is time well spent. Don't short-change yourself by cutting down on your hours of sleep. If possible, sleep outdoors. One night's rest outdoors is worth two indoors. And above all else—get away from noise."

What a character my grandfather was! Sleeping outside. Running around half-naked in the countryside. (Remember his advice on exercise?) I love that guy. He was a hippie way before I was, that's for sure.

Of course, times change. And, alas, few houses built today sport the open-air "sleeping porches" that were common in my grandfather's day, so the prospect of sleeping "outdoors" is a little more problematic now. What's more, the outdoors is considerably louder these days than it used to be, so sleeping out there probably isn't the best way to "get away from noise." But, though I can't second my grandfather's opinion that "one night's rest outdoors is worth two indoors," I can urge readers to seek ways to double the quality of their indoor sleep. That would make Grandpa proud, I hope.

My great-great-grandmother would be proud of me, too, I think. But in a different way. Ellen G. White was a notorious night owl, just like I am. Oh, she preached the importance of adequate rest. Don't get me wrong. In her *Testimonies for the Church, Volume 7* (1902), she wrote, "Proper periods of sleep and rest . . . are essential to health of body and mind. To rob nature of her hours for rest and recuperation . . . will result in irreparable loss."

But, truth be told, she didn't always practice what she preached. There are many stories in my family of how she would stay up half the night, or the whole night, writing letters or sermons or chapters of her latest book, and then transition with little or no rest into her usual strenuous workday.

I can't do that. I won't do that.

I don't need to do that.

After all, I don't have as big a job as she did. I'm not running a church. I don't write as prolifically as she felt called upon to do. And I don't have her superhuman powers.

I need my rest. And I have spent a lifetime learning how to get enough of it. I will share my secrets with you now.

- **EAT WELL.** There's no overstating the importance of this. If you'd like to experience the world's best sleep, give the world's best diet a try. Honestly, if you follow a plant-based whole foods meal plan, your body and mind will be happier, both in motion during the day and at rest during the night. I used to eat greasy foods, fatty foods, toxic foods, like most Americans do, and I used to wake up in the middle of the night with my guts on fire and a throat full of acid. My stomach would go sour during the day, too. I found myself buying antacids in those big warehouse-size jars and chewing them all the time. I kept a handful in my shirt pocket when I was out and about. And there were more in my car. And there were plenty more at home—in the kitchen, in the bathroom, and certainly in the bedroom, where those fiery wake-up calls became more and more frequent.

That's all in the past, though, it gives me joy to say. Now that I am eating better, I am living better and sleeping better. No more fire, no more acid. No more antacids.

- **GET SLEEPY.** A lot of people skip this step. They even fight it. They jack up themselves with late-night coffee. They pay bills or do other stressful things. They argue with their spouses. They turn on their computers and get themselves all worked up on the internet. Finally they go to bed, overstimulated and wide awake, and wonder why they have trouble falling asleep. Don't be like these people. I promise you, you will sleep much better if you go to bed ready to sleep. The secret is to treat your sleep time and your awake time with equal respect. Wear yourself out, in a good way, during your waking hours. Work hard, play hard, get enough exercise. Get good and tired. Then, retire. Power down. Get ready for bed, and then go to bed ready. Welcome sleep. It's the rest you've earned!

- **SLEEP NATURALLY.** Forcing yourself to sleep with pills or potions is a problem, not a solution. Sleeping pills can be unreliable, even ineffective, and definitely risky. They can produce unwanted side effects and result in dependency. I don't even like "natural" sleep-aid supplements like melatonin and valerian. I understand that some people find them helpful, but they don't work worth fiddlesticks on me. Even if they did offer some prospect of success, I would be concerned about using them. Popping a pill and waiting in anxious suspense for a miracle to happen is not a relaxing exercise for me.

- **TRY A NEW APPROACH.** You can't order yourself to sleep, so don't even try. There's no point in tossing and turning and twisting the night away, so stop it. If sleep won't come, get up for a bit. Do something quiet and calming. For example, sit in a comfortable chair and read by low lamplight. One of those thousand-page novels will do marvelously well. Haven't you always wanted to read *War and Peace*? Well, get started. I'm pretty sure you never will finish it, because you'll start dozing after a page or two. That's the idea!

- **RELAX.** If even *War and Peace* doesn't work, and you find yourself absolutely unable to fall asleep, don't sweat it. I mean this. Remind yourself that a state of restfulness is beneficial, even if it's not sleep. Accept it for what it is. Enjoy it. Take comfort in it. Think of all those times during a hectic day when you'd love to just close your eyes and rest for a minute. And, wow, here you are, getting to do just that! Feels good, doesn't it? Chances are, once you've taken the pressure off yourself, once you're relaxing contentedly instead of fretting and writhing about, your little half-doze will deepen into real sleep. See you in the morning!

I have a few relaxation tricks that I try on those pesky nights when sleep is a little slow to come. "Counting sheep" is not one of them. That works in cartoons, but it doesn't do much for me. Oh, I've tried it. I've mentally pictured sheep jumping over a fence, one by one, in endless succession. Trouble is, I'm not sure sheep are even capable of jumping over much of a fence, so pondering that implausibility always keeps me awake. Also, sheep make a lot of noise, baahing and braying the way they do, and they would make even more if they were trying to jump over a fence. Who can sleep with all that racket? Plus, if they did make it over the fence, they probably would poop when they landed on the other side. That is not a spectacle that will ever lull me into slumber.

No, I have other, better relaxation exercises.

I'll try taking slightly deeper breaths than usual. Sometimes I'll count them. More often than not, I'm asleep by sixty or seventy, though on occasion I've made it past one hundred. If that happens, I'll try something else.

I'll think of images that soothe me, usually broad landscapes, and I'll search for a pathway in them that will take me to the horizon.

Sometimes, as I drift off, I will be lifted into flight and I will view the scene from above as I soar over it.

I'll think of an old family photo, or perhaps a famous photo or painting, and I'll imagine myself entering the scene, where I can study the characters and the surroundings more closely, noting all the details down to the tiniest. It's as if I am diverting my attention from the real, waking world to an abstract "other" world. This is what falling asleep is all about, anyway, so it can be a very helpful exercise.

Sometimes, in the very last moments before I fall asleep, the characters and settings in the picture will come to life. The people will move and talk, and even turn to me, as if welcoming me to join their company. Sometimes this startles me back into full wakefulness and I lose the connection with the dream people. More often, though, I say yes to their invitation and join them in dreamland.

These transient visits to the weird place between wakefulness and sleep are certainly not unique to me. I may take an unusually active role in prompting them, by imagining scenes in my waking mind that then stir into action as my sleeping mind takes over, but there's nothing uncommon about the phenomenon itself. There's even a scientific term for it—hypnagogia. Author Kat Duff offers a fine discussion of it in her eloquent book *The Secret Life of Sleep* (Simon & Schuster/Atria Books/Beyond Words, 2014).

She writes, "During hypnagogia, clusters of neurons take turns shutting down, and sleep creeps over us. Our brain waves slow to a trance-like rhythm, and our attention drifts . . . People report fleeting visions of geometric patterns; sparks of light or splashes of color; and roaring, hissing, or clanging sounds . . . Occasionally, there is the sensation of floating, spinning, or getting bigger or smaller. It is a bizarre reality we slide through between waking and sleeping."

Let me tell you about one more mental relaxation trick of mine. And feel free to use it as inspiration for devising similar relaxation exercises of your own.

Instead of thinking about some old family photo, or some famous image, I start creating an imaginary picture of my own. It's a painting, and it's always the same one. I mentally pencil out a grid of equal, very small squares on a very large canvas. I locate the center square and, using an imaginary brush and an imaginary jar of paint, I mentally paint the square titanium white. I paint very carefully, keeping within the pencil lines. Next, I add a tiny drop of imaginary red paint to my jar of imaginary white paint and I carefully fill a square next to the first square. I add a second tiny drop of red paint to the white paint and use it to color the square below the second square. I continue this mental process, adding to the red content of the white paint in tiny increments and carefully, painstakingly filling squares in a clockwise whorl around the original square until there is perceptible, but only barely perceptible, evidence that the squares are reddening. Then, I mentally paint the next available square using a fresh jar of imaginary titanium white, then I start adding progressive drops of a different color, say yellow, to that white paint, continuing to enlarge the spiral of painted squares until the new color sequence becomes faintly evident. Then, there will be a third color sequence, and a fourth, and so on, until all the colors of the rainbow are seen, but only barely seen. My imaginary goal is to create a painting that seems at first glance to be a huge white checkerboard but with a phantom-like vortex of hinted other colors that flicker elusively within the whiteness of the whole.

Of course, my imaginary painting would be very calming, almost hypnotizing to view, just as it is very tranquilizing to create, and of course I never will finish it, because I usually am fast asleep not long after I start it. In fact, I usually nod off while I still am turning my first sequence of squares from bright white to vaguely pinkish. I never manage to even start the second sequence of colors!

I tell you, it's wearing me out just explaining this. In fact, I think I need to bring this chapter to a quick close.

I am getting sleepy.

I am getting so very, very sleepy.

A Happy Home Remedy for Insomnia

My Grandma Weeks raised her family alone on the hardscrabble flats of Texas and Arizona. She did right by her three children, Howard (my dad), Thelda, and Jean, and they all went on to great things.

Edith Weeks had a true frontierswoman's wisdom. I always loved listening to her stories, tall tales, jokes, and reminiscences. I remember she had a surefire cure for insomnia. She would eat a few cherries before bed. She liked them sour, too! They kept her regular and helped her sleep, she said.

I've checked, by the way, and there actually is some science to support my grandmother's homespun notion. Cherries are a rare natural food source of melatonin, the hormone in the human body that helps regulate sleeping and waking cycles. The melatonin found in most drugs and nutritional supplements is a manufactured synthetic.

CHAPTER FIFTEEN

Dream Well

IF I EVER MANAGE TO FIGURE OUT WHAT DREAMS ARE ALL ABOUT, I WILL GO RENT an apartment in Stockholm and start writing my Nobel Prize acceptance speech.

We humans have solved so many other mysteries. We have discovered so much. We have invented, cured, created, and conquered. We have overcome one obstacle after another in understanding and tapping the potential of what we humans are capable of doing.

While we're awake.

But what do we make of our other lives, the ones we lead while we are asleep?

The scenes in that other reality can be so vivid, the actions so dramatic, the stories so simmering with portent, and yet we know almost nothing about that place or the meaning of what takes place there. We are essentially clueless.

Although we have extended almost boundlessly the reach of our waking selves, our working knowledge of dreams and dreaming has not advanced at all during the whole course of human history. Indeed, we may know and understand even less about them than did our distant ancestors, who seem to have taken their dreams quite seriously and literally. Their literature is full of examples. Dreams are a powerful driver of the narrative in works ranging from the Bible to Greek mythology to Arthurian legend.

If, alas, I never do figure out what dreams are all about, and never do have the occasion to write and deliver that gracious speech in Stockholm, it will not be for lack of trying. I have made it a lifetime effort.

As a very young child, not even school age, I dreamed often of the Devil. Finally, the nightmares became too much for me. I warned Satan in no uncertain terms that he was running a serious risk. I told him that if he continued to plague me in my dreams, he would convince me of his real-life existence. Furthermore, I told him, once I became convinced that he was real, I naturally would conclude beyond doubt that God, his opposite, is also real. And, happy in that knowledge, I would embrace God unreservedly. Thank you, Satan, I would say to him, for neatly proving the existence of God and making my choice an easy one. By your own actions, Satan, I would say to him, you have lost the battle for my soul!

And thus did I checkmate the Devil. He has not troubled me since. Apparently, he still is embarrassed at being outmaneuvered by a youngster.

It's not surprising that I would possess a hardwired interest in dreams, given that I am directly descended from Ellen G. White, famous for her dreams and visions. Of course, hers were prophetic and instructive. They were foundational in the building of a global religious movement and health ministry that continues to thrive and grow today.

My dreams are not prophetic. Believe me, my one crack at the prophecy game was a laughable failure. Once, during a year I was living in Europe and working on my master's degree, I had a dream that my father had died. It was so lucid and forceful, I was sure it was a divination of a real event. There was no phone in my rented flat, so I walked hurriedly to the nearby village square and used a pay phone. International calls were a real ordeal in those days, so it took me forever to get through.

Finally, though, I could hear the phone ringing in Loma Linda, California, six thousand miles away.

My dad answered.

"Hello?" he said, in his booming baritone voice.

He was fine.

Never better.

He lived in perfect health for another forty years.

No, my dreams are not prophetic.

Most of the time, they aren't even special. I've had this one dream my whole life, and I used to think it was a big deal. I call it my "school dream" and I still have it, though my school days are long past. The dream has several variations, but the theme never varies. There's a big test tomorrow, or a big paper due, and I haven't even started preparing for it. Or else I suddenly will realize, in my dream, that I haven't even been to class in ages. I have fallen impossibly behind. How am I ever going to graduate?

This recurring "school dream" is very stressful, and I used to think it had profound meaning. I always would wake up relieved, of course, because in real life there were no tests or papers or other class requirements hanging over my head. My graduation was a done deal. Still, I would be troubled by what I took to be the message of my dream: I must be falling behind schedule in accomplishing my goals, and failing to meet my expectations for myself.

Then, about a year ago, I was reading *Parade* magazine in the Sunday newspaper and I almost fell out of my chair when I came across the "Ask Marilyn" column by Marilyn vos Savant. It featured a letter from one of her readers who described a recurring "school dream" exactly like mine.

I almost fell out of my chair again when the columnist answered by saying she often had the same dream herself.

Then, a few weeks later, I almost fell out of my chair again when she reported in a follow-up column that "hundreds" of readers had written in to say that they, too, have that identical recurring dream.

There's more. Just recently I was reading and enjoying an excellent book titled *Dreamland: Adventures in the Strange Science of Sleep* (Norton, 2013), by journalist David K. Randall. And, son of a gun, *he's* had that dream, too!

Yes, I almost fell out of my chair again.

OK, so my dreams aren't always special. I admit it.

But they often are entertaining. Sometimes they are even useful. I always, always pay attention to them.

One night in 1977 I dreamed that I was interviewing people in a huge line that snaked around the Superdome in New Orleans. There was much excitement. A Beatles reunion concert had been announced and the rush for tickets was itself a news-making event. Television helicopters patrolled the sky. On the ground, a large security force labored to maintain crowd control.

This was a time when all four Beatles were still alive. They had disbanded only a few years previously and wild rumors of their coming together again seemed always to be in circulation, though all four of them were adamant it never would happen.

Intrigued by my dream, I developed and wrote a whole fictional story around it that involved the Beatles being kidnapped and forced to perform a spectacular concert, against their will, in order to regain their freedom. In my story, the compulsory rehearsals for this gig are bitter and acrimonious, of course, as the Beatles rage not only against their abductors but also against each other. Something wonderful happens, though, when they finally take the Superdome stage and start to play. The magic of their songs and the adoration of their fans take hold and turn the concert by degrees into a jubilant event that exhilarates the crowd and the Beatles both.

My story was published internationally, so I'm not giving anything away by telling you the ending. We learn that the abductors were only actors and the whole kidnapping was a staged affair. Arranged and financed by Ringo!

Yes, it was Ringo Starr who wanted more than anything else to get the band together one last time. In the story, he confesses all during a tearful hug-out with his bandmates following the show.

Playboy magazine purchased my story for a nice four-figure sum. Titled "The Beatles' Not-So-Magical Mystery Tour," it appeared in the March 1978 issue of *Oui* magazine, a *Playboy* subsidiary of that era. It later appeared, in Spanish translation, in the South American edition of *Playboy* itself.

There was immense reaction to the story. Letters to the editor appeared for months afterward. Among those offering comment were Olivia Harrison, wife of George, and the actress Barbara Bach, wife of Ringo. They both loved the story, they said, though Ringo's wife insisted he never would have done such a thing!

A big-shot Hollywood producer tracked me down and offered me big bucks and a consulting editor credit for a movie inspired by my story. Ultimately, it didn't work out, for various reasons, but it was a thrill ride for a while. I was invited to a gala announcement party at a Los Angeles hotel where there was much hoopla. There was even a rumor that George Harrison might drop by!

He never did, but my seatmate during our fancy catered meal was Mitch Weissman, who was playing the role of Paul McCartney in the new smash Broadway musical *Beatlemania*, so that was plenty enough excitement for me.

Oh, and there was more in store. Almost fifteen years later, I was tickled to learn that my old short story had earned a mention in a hot new book of almost 500 pages, *The Ultimate Beatles Quiz Book* by Michael J. Hockinson (St. Martin's Griffin, 1992). Believe me, it's a thrill to find your name in a book about the Beatles!

Remember, all of this happened because of a simple dream.

I'm a writer, so I often dream in story form. Other kinds of people have other kinds of dreams. Athletes have sports dreams. Scientists have science dreams. Engineers dream of building things.

Jack Nicklaus in 1964 literally dreamed up a small trick for fine-tuning his golf swing, which resulted in one of the great careers in the history of the sport and put many millions of dollars into his pocket. James Watson, co-discoverer in 1953 of the double helix structure of DNA, attributed his inspiration to a dream about a spiral staircase. Albert Einstein said that various images from his dream life in the early 1900s helped inform his theory of relativity. Elias Howe invented the sewing machine in 1845 after a dream of cannibals brandishing threaded spears.

You see, dreams can have practical value. It's something to consider for all you dreamers out there. Let me offer a little additional illustration from my own experience.

In 1990, a new television drama titled *Twin Peaks* became an international phenomenon. It was such a big deal that *Time* magazine featured executive producer and director David Lynch on its cover. The show was a surreal murder mystery set in a woodsy community where nothing was what it seemed and everyone had a secret. A homecoming queen was found murdered and the list of suspects grew longer with each week's episode. Millions of viewers tuned in to ABC each week, hoping for an answer to the big question: Who killed Laura Palmer?

I was a big fan. One night, very early on in the show's run, I had a dream. A large crowd had formed around me and there were horrified looks on their faces. I was mortified, too. I had just blurted out a confession. I killed Laura Palmer! The crowd around me tightened. It was about to become an angry mob bent on vengeance. I was surrounded. I didn't stand a chance.

That's when I woke, terrified, my heart racing.

I had that "whew-it-was-only-a-dream" moment. I chuckled. I shook it off. But, then, I couldn't get it out of my mind.

I thought about that dream all day. And it inspired me with an idea. In the world of dreams, where a fictional murder can seem real, my confession had felt awful, and the crowd response chilling. In the real world, though, a confession to a fictional killing would be recognized as a joke, right? The big crowd response would be to laugh, right?

Right?

I called a friend that evening, a *Twin Peaks* fan like me, and asked him what he thought might happen if I got a bunch of T-shirts printed up with the words: "I KILLED LAURA PALMER." He laughed, then thought a moment, and said, "People would buy those."

I followed through. I spent a little money having a couple dozen T-shirts made at a local silk-screening shop and, sure enough, I sold all of them in no time to friends and colleagues at the newspaper where I worked. It was an immediate doubling of my investment.

Word spread. I started hearing from friends at other newspapers around Southern California. I went and had more shirts made.

Columnists at those other newspapers started mentioning the "I KILLED LAURA PALMER" T-shirts in their columns, and I then started hearing from the public. I went and had more shirts made.

Pretty soon columnists at newspapers all over the country were mentioning my shirts, and I was receiving orders by the armload. I went and had more shirts made. Lots more.

I was featured on local television. Then, national television. I appeared on the CBS show *Entertainment Tonight*, in a segment introduced by anchor Mary Hart, that aired on August 13, 1990. The segment even included a cut-away interview with David Lynch himself, who gave the whole thing his good-natured blessing. "It's a good thing that those T-shirts came about," he said. "It's fine with me."

Of course, at about the same time, I also received a sternly worded cease-and-desist letter from his production company. The folks there had decided that the apparent demand for *Twin Peaks* merchandise should be fulfilled by them, not me.

It was OK. I complied immediately. I had enjoyed my fun. I had made quite a few thousand dollars. I had gotten my face on network television. It was all good.

And all of this happened because of a ten-second dream of mine. (Who knows, maybe *Twin Peaks* itself happened as the result of a ten-second dream in the fascinating head of David Lynch!) The moral of the story is this: Pay attention to those ten-second dreams. Some of them are good ones. And you know what? The more attention you pay to them, the more of them you're likely to have, and the more likely you are to remember them.

Here's another thing you can do to improve your dream life. Eat the world's best diet! Seriously. What's good for your body is good for your brain, and what's good for your brain is good for your dreams.

A plant-based whole foods diet of fresh fruits, vegetables, leafy greens, whole grains, nuts, seeds, and legumes promotes not only physical health but also mental health. You can have a body that performs like a champ while you're awake, and a brain that performs like a champ while you're asleep.

Eat well, sleep well, dream well.

I used to wake up often from upsetting dreams and find that my body was upset, too. I had fire in my guts and acid in my throat. I had a headache and a raging thirst.

Too much rich, greasy food. Too much strong drink. Not enough water.

My body was sputtering on bad fuel, which distressed my brain, which disturbed my sleep. And my dreams.

I've put those days (and nights) behind me. Now, I'm eating good food and drinking plenty of clean, cold water. My body's engine runs better during the day while I'm awake, and it idles better at night while I'm asleep. That means better sleep and better dreams.

It's cause and effect, and it can work as well for you as it does for me. You should try it.

I'll tell one more story, to further illustrate the point of this chapter. It's a story with roots in one decade and literary results in two others.

Some time in the 1980s, I dreamed I was hiking on the Vivian Creek Trail that heads up out of the San Bernardino Mountains community of Forest Falls, not far from my home, and climbs all the way to San Gorgonio Peak—the loftiest elevation in Southern California. I have hiked this trail a thousand times, and I also dream about it often.

In this dream, I was traversing Vivian Creek Meadow that lies in heavy shadow in a deep cut between two ramparts of the mountain, about a mile up the trail. It is always dark here, as high forest grows and overhangs it on both sides, but in this dream I became fascinated by a brilliant light that glowed through the trees on one of the hillcrests far above me.

Believe me, in real life I do not leave the designated trail when hiking in the wilderness, and I advise all you boys and girls not to do it either, but this was a dream, and I left the trail in search of that light.

My course led up and over the hillcrest into a strange new wildland with forbidding tangles of thorny manzanita and sudden precipices that would open upon dizzying chasms that fell out of view far below. I struggled over huge boulders and through long tunnels of dirt and rock as I made my way higher and higher into this new, strange frontier.

Finally, I broke free into a broad clearing that widened to the edge of a huge canyon that fell away beyond it. Eagles flew in great numbers above the abyss. On the far edge of the clearing upon which I stood, where the ground gave way to the void, there was a small hut. I approached and tried the door. It opened. There was nothing inside except a door in the opposite wall that I knew could lead only to one thing, the open sky full of eagles and the plummeting depths below.

With feelings of both elation and dread, I approached that door and put out my hand to open it. I was covered with goosebumps. My hair was standing on end.

Then I woke up. And, yes, I was covered with goosebumps. And my hair was standing on end.

That was the end of my dream, but it wasn't the end of the short story I proceeded to write based on that dream. In the story, which I titled "A Door in the Mountains," there's an extended finale. I find much and learn much in that little hut. I meet someone who reveals the secret of the second door and the importance of the eagles. I won't tell you how it ends because I still have hopes of publishing it one day.

I almost got it published then.

I sent it to *Outside* magazine, which was fairly new at the time. I heard back from one of the editors there. He loved the story and wanted to buy it, but other editors there objected. It was not a literary magazine. Publishing a piece of fiction would set a dangerous precedent. The other editors didn't want to go in that direction.

The one editor kept encouraging me. He continued to fight for it for many months and he reported back to me several times, telling me to have patience.

It never came to anything. Apparently, the one editor lost his battle with the other editors because I stopped hearing from him and, by then, I was involved in several other projects, so I stopped thinking about "A Door in the Mountains."

For about twenty years.

Then, during the first decade of the new century, while working on a novel in collaboration with a longtime friend and fellow journalist, my memories of that old story were stirred. I dug it out of my filing cabinet and read it again. Yes, I could use portions of it in the novel. After all, our novel's main character and his girlfriend make a miraculous discovery when they go off-trail in the San Gorgonio Wilderness. Pretty similar detail.

So, parts of the old short story based on a dream became parts of the novel *Window Beyond the World*, by John Howard Weeks and William S. Thomas, published in 2006.

And, wait, there's more! An essay I wrote about the collaborative effort that Bill and I undertook in writing that book ended up in another book, *Choice Words: The Borgo Press Book of Writers Writing About Writing*, published by Wildside Press in 2010. My essay is chapter fourteen, titled "The Two-Headed Author."

So, abracadabra, that's another example of how a little dream of mine has yielded tangible results in my wide-awake life.

What I hope is that these anecdotes serve to make a point. Dreams matter.

For anyone, I believe. Maybe your own dreams won't yield story plots, or golf tips, or new scientific theories, or important new inventions, but they may yield any number of other things of value, if you pay attention.

A dream might help you identify sources of stress in your life, which might then put you on the path toward resolving those issues. A dream might help you clarify your ideas about a situation that challenges you. A dream might help you look at a relationship in a new way. A dream can trigger ideas, point to opportunities, prompt a course change, or offer a new perspective on matters great and small.

Many people claim they never remember their dreams, but that's because they never take notice of them. Once you start taking note, I promise you, you'll notice more and more.

It's not like you have to bolt upright in your bed each morning and write furiously in a dream diary, although I personally envy those who do that. Psychologist Carl Jung and novelist Jack Kerouac kept dream diaries, and the practice served them well. They had some pretty terrific dreams.

Here's what I do when a particular dream strikes my fancy. I scribble a little note about it on a piece of scrap paper and throw it into the drawer of my bedside table. That helps me keep it in mind for a while, which helps determine its impact on me. If I soon forget all about it, well, OK, it was forgettable. If it still is popping up in my head days later, well, I start considering the possibility that it's a keeper, and perhaps I should make something of it. I go back to the bedside drawer, fish out the note, and read it again.

Believe me, that drawer is full of future stories and novels and other books. I will have to live a long, long time to write them all.

Like I said at the beginning of this chapter, the phenomenon of dreaming is near the top of the list of things that fascinate me. What are dreams? How do they happen? What do they mean?

It took me years of thinking about my dreams to realize that there is usually, if not always, an unseen companion in my dream narratives. I feel his presence. I converse with him. I act in unison with him. But I never quite see him. I see all the other people in my dreams, face to face, but never this one steady companion at my side.

I finally decided, and I don't know whether it was a realization or a guess, that this other person is . . . me.

He is my double. There are two of us.

One of us lives in my dream world and the other one of us lives in my waking world, and the two of us hook up when I fall asleep.

Of course, I only can speak for my waking self. My dream self might have a very different opinion about who does what, and when.

Who is this other John? Is he my soul? My angel? My ghost?

Or maybe he's my brain, who never sleeps. He continues to romp around while I, his weaker half, his physical half, weary of bone and body, take my necessary rest. I can understand why he might get impatient at times, even bored, and always ready to welcome me when I slip into my dream gear and join him on his adventures. He always has the craziest places he wants to go, and the craziest stuff he wants to show me.

One of these nights, I hope he shows me, or tells me, what dreams are all about. That would be so awesome. If he does, I promise you'll be hearing from me.

In fact, everyone will be hearing from me.

I will be addressing the world from Stockholm.

A Happy Home Remedy for Nightmares

Long ago, sage was used to cast out evil spirits. The potent herb still is used in Native American "smudging" ceremonies to remove negative energy from a room or other space. Sage also has many uses in natural medicine. Herbalists recommend it as a calming natural sedative that helps relieve stress, anxiety, insomnia, and sleep disorders, including night terrors and nightmares.

For anyone suffering from troublesome dreams, it might be worth a shot to keep a supply of herbal sage tea around the house. It's available in bulk or tea bag form at health food stores and online.

Sip a steaming cup of sage tea before bedtime, and then fall asleep with confidence. Trust the power!

CHAPTER SIXTEEN

Good Morning, Merry Sunshine

I'VE HAD A LIFELONG LOVE AFFAIR WITH THE SUN.

Things have gotten pretty hot and steamy between us.

That's why I always use protection.

Yes, you should see my impressive collection of sun hats. And I have lots of long-sleeve shirts that are loose and lightweight and well-ventilated enough to wear even in summer. When I must use sunscreen I choose products that have an SPF (Sun Protection Factor) of at least 40, often more.

I live in sunny Southern California, less than an hour's drive from some of the most beautiful and famous beaches on Earth.

But I am no beach bum.

Oh, I visit beach towns all the time, because I love the sort of shops and art galleries and cafés that are to be found there. But you will never find me lying on a towel in the sand, working on my suntan.

For one thing, having my body coated with a greasy, gritty combination of sunscreen lotion, sweat, and sand is not my idea of comfort or pleasure.

Also, and more importantly, I am smart enough to know that a suntan is a skin injury. A sunburn is a severe skin injury. Skin damage can lead to wrinkles, disfigurement, cancer, and death.

I see the Beautiful People baking in oil on a hot beach and I think, "Fools, you will die young. And ugly."

In ancient times, it was the poor classes, the peasants, obliged to labor outdoors, who had sun-weathered skin. The rich people, the beautiful people of the time, went to extremes to keep their skin fair and unblemished by the elements.

Peons had great tans. Lords and ladies looked like ghosts.

Today, it's quite the other way around. The laborers who work outdoors have enough sense to wear sun protection, while the rich and famous lie poolside or at the beach, barbecuing themselves to a bubbly brown.

This complete reversal is just one more example of how history often does not follow a sensible straight line.

I've had two sunburns in my entire life. I hated them so much that I vowed never to have one again. I fell asleep on a beach once when I was a kid. And I fell asleep by a swimming pool once when I was a teenager. Both times I turned as red as a roast, which was ugly indeed. Then I started molting and shedding my skin, which was even uglier. Hellish fever turned to horrid itchiness. I writhed against walls like a bear against trees, trying to scratch my scorched back. My face looked like a mummy's on a bad day.

I did not feel like one of the Beautiful People.

Now, please, don't get me wrong. Sunshine is wonderful.

In moderation.

It's one of the Nature's Seven Doctors featured in the 1962 book of that title co-written by my grandfather, Herbert C. White. (And, since we've covered most of the seven by now, let's review. They are "fresh air," "good food," "pure water," "sunshine," "exercise," "rest," and "power of the mind.")

"Sunshine is the most marvelous health-giving and healing power in all the world," my grandfather wrote. "It is heaven's free gift to man. Old and young should spend several hours each day in the open air and the sunshine."

He himself spent as much time as possible outdoors, tending his gardens, digging in the dirt, working his compost piles, so he certainly did practice his own preaching. But he took care, too. He was a fair-skinned man, descended from Northern European stock, and he was mindful of the dangers of overexposure to the sun.

I never saw him working in his garden without a hat on his head. Indeed, some of his hats were such outlandish, bonnet-style creations, I still giggle when I think of them.

My grandfather's collaborator, Dr. H. E. Kirschner, was more daring. I didn't know him, but many of the photographs I have seen of him show a fearless sort of sun worship on his part. In fact, there are two such photos of Dr. Kirschner in *Nature's Seven Doctors*. One shows a wintry scene of about 1910 outside a tuberculosis hospital called the Pennsylvania Sanitorium, located in Kirschner's home state. The young doctor is seen with three of his patients, all of them basking in the midwinter sun, seated on recliner chairs set out in the snow. The three patients, all of them women, are wearing hats. Dr. Kirschner is not. He squints amiably with full sunshine on his face.

As any skier will tell you, the magnified impact of reflected sunshine on snow can pose a real threat of sunburn.

The other picture, taken a decade later, after Dr. Kirschner moved to Southern California, shows a bright summery scene at his home in Monrovia, a little northeast of Los Angeles. Wearing only a loincloth, he lies baking on a hospital-style bed that has been set up on his sun porch. His skin glistens with perspiration. It's a black-and-white photograph so, mercifully, if he is lobster-red, we cannot see it.

Dr. Kirschner was irrepressible in his praise of the therapeutic benefits of sunbathing. He was fond of saying to his patients, "Where fresh air and sunshine enter little, the doctor enters often."

Listen to this story of his, told in *Nature's Seven Doctors*:

"It was during my visit to Switzerland that I received a very striking lesson on the superlative value of sunshine, not only to the sick and afflicted, but to an entire population, as well. In the deep valleys among the Alps the sun shines only a few hours each day. In consequence, the inhabitants suffer terribly from scrofula and other diseases . . . Many of the women suffer from goiters, and many of the males are idiots. But strange as it may seem, higher up on the sunny slopes of the mountains the inhabitants are remarkably hardy and are well developed both physically and mentally. The only difference in their modes of life is the greater amount of sunshine at the higher altitudes. When the sick, unfortunate ones who live in the deep valleys are brought up the mountainside, with longer daily exposure to the healing rays of the sun, they rapidly improve."

There's another story in the same chapter, and this one comes from my grandfather, and it involves my own family. It's only summarized in the book, but I heard it in expanded form, on many occasions, from my grandfather's own lips. It's a story about his grandmother, my great-great-grandmother.

In 1900, when Ellen G. White and her family returned to America after a prolonged residence in sunny Australia, where they did extensive missionary work, they lived for a while in rented quarters situated in a dark ravine between two prodigious hills in California's Napa County, north of San Francisco. The lack of sunshine at that location became a source of complaint when the family was beset by a seemingly endless succession of colds, fevers, and infections. After they bought their own home, called Elmshaven, in a much sunnier part of Napa Valley near the town of St. Helena, the family's good health returned.

Ellen G. White was a great believer in the healthful effects of sunshine. "Go out into the light and warmth of the glorious sun," she wrote. "Share its life-giving, healing power" (*The Health Reformer*, 1871).

She also believed in having plenty of sunlight indoors, which was quite a departure from the fashion of the day, ruled by the Victorian penchant for dark, airless, heavily draped interiors.

"If you would have your homes sweet and inviting, make them bright with air and sunshine," she wrote in *Counsels on Health*, published posthumously in 1923. "Remove the heavy curtains, open the windows, throw back the blinds, and enjoy the rich sunlight, even if it be at the expense of the color of your carpets. The precious sunlight may fade your carpets, but it will give healthful color to the cheeks of your children. A home made bright with air and sunlight, and cheerful with the welcome of unselfish hospitality, will be a heaven below!"

Today, we know all about the sun's salubrious effects on our bodies and spirits. We also know about the hazards of immoderate exposure to the sun. We know so much, in fact, that we have no excuse not to be smart consumers of sunshine.

Here are tips I've collected over the years from various sources, including my own family lore.

- **RUB-A-DUB-DUB.** If you're like most sensible people, you know it's important to apply sunscreen lotion to all parts of your body that will be exposed to the sun for more than a few minutes. But make sure you're using the right stuff and using enough of it. Choose a broad spectrum UVA-UVB sunscreen that offers an SPF of at least 30. I remember when 15 was considered OK, but it's double that now, and many dermatologists recommend 40, 50, even 60, depending on skin type, length of exposure, and other factors.

   OK, once you've got the right stuff, slather it on generously. Get the fronts of both hands good and wet with lotion, then rub it into your face and neck. Do the same thing for other areas of your body that need sun protection. On a swimsuit day, that means not only your face and ears and neck but also your shoulders, arms, tummy and chest, back, upper legs, lower legs, and feet. That's eight big squirts of sunscreen lotion.
- **WHO'S GOT YOUR BACK?** Unless you're a contortionist, you can't rub your own back. If you don't have a friend to help, use a spray-form sunscreen. A spray is fine. Not nearly as fun as a friend, though.
- **KEEP UP THE GOOD WORK.** Sun protection isn't a once-and-done deal. You should reapply sunscreen every couple of hours, and always after swimming or towel drying.

- **YOU SAY YOU DON'T LIKE SUNSCREEN?** Fine. There are other ways to cover up. Wear loose, lightweight, well-ventilated clothing that provides sufficient sun protection. And put on a hat. I don't mean a baseball cap. I mean a wide-brimmed hat that completely shades your face and neck. They are available in every imaginable style. Find one that looks good on you. Or, if you like to make little kids giggle, find one of those big, crazy ones like my grandfather used to wear.

- **LIP SERVICE.** When I apply sunscreen lotion to my face, I try to avoid getting it in my mouth. I find that I don't like the taste. But does this mean that my lips are left unprotected from the sun? Good heavens, no! I would not let that happen. Cancer of the lip is a particularly nasty one. No, thank you. What I do, and what you should do, is use a good lip balm that offers sunscreen protection. I carry a stick in my pocket at all times. I could just say ChapStick, because that's what it is, but I would be embarrassed if the ChapStick company feels it must send me a huge check in exchange for my endorsement. I will respect their decision, however.

- **DON'T LET LUBRICATION TAKE A VACATION.** Sunscreen and moisturizing lotion are not the same thing. People forget that. And some people stop using moisturizing lotion in warm weather. They figure, hey, they're using sunscreen instead. And they're sweating, which makes them feel juiced up.

  They're fooling themselves. Sweat is moisture leaving the body, not moisture coming in. Sweating calls for more moisturizing, not less. And sunscreen is not a substitute for moisturizer. Sunscreen protects the surface of your skin from the sun's ultraviolet rays, but it doesn't penetrate and replenish dry skin the way a good moisturizer will do.

  Dry skin is a year-round concern, so it's important to maintain your moisturizing routine—summer, winter, spring, and fall.

- **INSIDER INFORMATION.** Guess what? Good skin care doesn't just happen on the outside. You can do wonders for your skin by nourishing it from the inside, too. It's simple. Just drink plenty of water (see chapter nine, "The World's Best Beverage") and eat lots of fruits and vegetables (see chapter four, "The World's Best Diet"). Water refreshes all your organs, including your skin. And food nutrients that are rich in phytochemicals are as good for your skin as they are for the rest of you. Studies show that lycopene, found in tomatoes and other red fruits and vegetables, can help protect skin from the sun's damaging ultraviolet rays. Carotenoids, the disease-fighting antioxidants found in orange and yellow fruits and vegetables, are helpful in the same way. Cruciferous vegetables, such as broccoli, cauliflower, Brussels sprouts, kale, cabbage, and bok choy, are abundant with cancer-busting glucosinolates and other phytochemicals that will help keep your skin in tip-top shape.

  You're going to find a lot of terrific recipes for dishes just bursting with this stuff in chapter twenty-one of this book: Creamy Broccoli Salad with broccoli, Triple Slaw with cabbage, Monkey-Bunny Cake with carrots, Mediterranean Wheat Salad with yellow squash, Pizza Allegro with orange and red and yellow bell peppers, and Three Amigos Chili with lots of tomatoes. Those are just a few of many examples. Coming right up!

A Happy Home Remedy for Sunburn

We've talked about stuff you can use to save yourself from overexposure to the sun. But what if you screw up? What if, in spite of all the good advice, you forget to use that stuff, or you don't use enough, and you end up with a sunburn? Is there stuff you can use then? Yes. I recommend aloe vera. The spiky succulent plant is filled with gel that offers wonderful natural relief for minor sunburn, as well as insect bites and other skin irritations. I grow several aloe vera plants in my garden year-round. They are hardy plants that can be cultivated indoors in pots, too. Any time I get a little kitchen burn I will run out, break off a good chunk of one of the spikes, and rub the clear gel on my wound. Instant relief! Aloe vera gel is also available in commercial preparations to be found at pharmacies and health food stores. Some people use aloe vera as part of their daily moisturizing routine. It's good stuff.

CHAPTER SEVENTEEN

The Straight Poop

I USED TO HAVE A RATHER IRRITABLE BOWEL, BUT ITS MOOD IS MUCH IMPROVED of late, thanks very much.

Sometimes I think I was actually born with irritable bowel syndrome, and I think a lot of other people might say the same, if they allowed themselves to speak of such indelicate matters.

Think about it. Doctors for generations made it a practice to slap newborn babies on the bottom to make them cry. Supposedly, the spanking would kick-start the respiratory system and put infants on their way to breathing independently.

But maybe that slap on the butt did something else, too. Maybe a lot of us started our lives feeling a little cranky about what goes on down there.

And, sometimes, things that start badly keep getting worse.

Parents apply a lot of psychological pressure, I believe. They try to potty train their kids as soon as possible. Or even sooner than possible. Then, when the kids are potty trained, they are pressured to use the bathroom on their parents' schedule, not their own.

I remember being marched to the bathroom all the time and being told to poop "right now," so we wouldn't be late for this or that. On car trips we would stop for bathroom breaks when the folks decided the time was right. That was great for them. They were ready to perform.

For us kids, who maybe weren't quite ready to perform, well, that was too bad. We missed our chance.

We were S.O.L., which stands for you-know-what outta luck.

Pressure to perform one's doody on demand can do a real number on a child's system. And, no, when I say "do a real number," I don't mean No. 2, because No. 2 is a good thing, not a bad thing. Here's the bad thing: Parental pressure on a child's bathroom behavior can lead to long-lasting physical afflictions including constipation, retention, gas and bloat, abdominal pain, irritable bowel, hemorrhoids, and more, plus myriad emotional woes, including anxiety, panic, dread, and self-loathing.

When I was a kid, I acted out in the bathroom in many ways. One of them was so peculiar that it makes me laugh today to think about it, though it's one of those rueful laughs that leaves a pained look on my face.

When Mom or Dad decided it was time for me to poop, and shooed me into the bathroom, whether at home or on the road, they would wait outside for my command performance to proceed. What I did first was to remove every stitch of clothing, including my socks and underpants. Even if it was an outdoor public toilet in the middle of a freezing cold park in the dead of winter, I would end up barefoot and buck naked, standing there in the stall, staring warily at the toilet, contemplating the task before me with dread and misgiving.

I'm not sure why the clothes had to come off. Maybe I thought that ungirding my body would get me "in the mood" to perform this awful bodily obligation. More likely, it was just something to do to keep busy while I passed the time in there, not daring to come out until a sufficient number of minutes had passed.

Believe me, minutes were usually the only things that were passed during these ordeals. I would sit on the toilet, obediently, and strain and grunt, and strain and grunt some more, then I would go through the motions of using the tissue dispenser and flushing the toilet in order to make all the appropriate noises for my eager audience outside to hear. Then I would get dressed and walk out, my dismal charade completed. I would look into the expectant eyes of Mom or Dad or both, then compound the sin of not pooping with the sin of lying about it.

"Did you go doo-doo?" I would be asked.

"Yes," I would testify falsely.

"That's a good boy," I would be told, with a pat on my head.

I know there are legions of others in the world who grew up scarred by the hard knocks of potty training and toilet tyranny. I know that even as adults they continue to suffer performance anxiety and dysfunction. I know, because I find it necessary now and then to visit public restrooms and I hear the futile exertions of these sufferers in nearby stalls. They remind me of myself as a boy, though presumably they haven't stripped themselves naked from head to toe, as I used to do.

If they have, I don't want to know about it.

I also observe that there is a booming laxative industry, with reported sales of nearly $1 billion each year in the United States alone, so I know it's not just my imagination telling me that many, many poor souls are obliged to endure the companionship of bowels that are traumatized and noncompliant. Irritable, to say the least.

Fortunately, there are natural remedies that are immediately available and effective, including diet and meditation exercises, as I soon will explain. (And if anyone is lifting an eyebrow at the mention of meditation, let me assert emphatically that contemplating one's bowel is no more unusual than contemplating one's navel. They aren't that far apart.)

First, though, before I begin to share these particulars, I want to make a little speech on why I think that a well-working bowel is a key to good health and long life.

I sometimes am shocked to hear actual medical doctors say that it is quite OK to not have a bowel movement every day. I even have heard it said that an entire week without a bowel movement is not a matter for alarm. I almost faint when I hear such reckless talk. If I held back on my poop for an entire week, then let it go all at once, I first would have to file an environmental impact statement with the city. Maybe the whole county. I don't know how many communities would be endangered.

Of course, I never would wait a week to poop. I won't wait a single day.

Poop is a waste product. It needs proper, prompt disposal. It can't be allowed to sit around and rot and fester and ferment.

If you are storing your waste instead of eliminating it, you are poisoning your body. Here's a comparison: A backed-up sewer system can make a whole building uninhabitable. A backed-up digestive system can have a similar effect on your body.

I no longer wonder at all the people I see, every day, who look stricken and miserable. I used to think they were carrying the weight of the world upon their shoulders. Now I know it's the weight of something else, somewhere else.

Balky bowels are a big problem. But fixing the problem is no big deal. You can start today. First, stop eating so much meat. The bodies of those poor animals that you are sticking into your own body are hanging around to haunt you. I'll put it another way. If you take in a lot of dead stuff at the top end, you'll end up with a lot of dead weight at your bottom end.

Try eating more fruits, vegetables, nuts, beans, and other high-fiber foods and you'll notice a difference right away. You won't have to strain to squeeze out old hardened stools that stink to high heaven. No, you'll feel your system moving things along at an exhilarating clip. Your poop will be loose, lubed, easy to unload. And it will have a fresh, springtime scent!

OK, I am exaggerating about that last bit. But honestly, you'll soon notice you aren't using as much room deodorant as you once did. Me, I never use the stuff. Don't need it.

If my friends tell you any differently, they are jealous lying bastards.

As long as we are talking about the smell of poop, let me mention another sensitive issue, and that is the appearance of poop. I've heard it said by responsible people speaking in respectable forums—or wait a minute, maybe it was just a bunch of crazy folks jabbering away on

TV talk shows—that your poop ideally should land in the toilet in the form of the letter C.

I may have heard that the letter S is acceptable, too.

Hey, maybe the letter Q would be best, because that would mean you have pooped enough to form a complete circle, then added an extra squiggle for good measure!

Nonsense. I don't agree with people who say we should poop alphabet letters.

In fact, I think these people are full of . . . no, I won't say it.

But I will say this. If your poop has any firm shape at all, it is too dry and compacted. This means it has been in your system too long.

Good poop should have a loose, fall-apart consistency. It should be almost formless. It should look like roughage in your toilet, not alphabet letters as hard as sausages.

That's my opinion, and it took me years of sitting and thinking about it before I knew I was right.

Historically, mankind has made a sorry business of doing its business. We have allowed our bowels to vex us for too long.

Believe me, I've heard stories.

I've heard of tribal people in primitive times who would prepare their virgins for marriage by stuffing them with a banquet of foods, then sending in the female elders to work the virgin over with abdominal palpations to move the food through and out in time for the wedding. Or, wait, maybe this was how they prepared their virgins for sacrifice to the volcano gods. Anyway, it was a real ordeal.

I've heard of ancient monks who would attempt to stimulate their bowels by swallowing a thick knotted string tied at one end to a tooth. When the other end of the string worked its way through the intestines and out the back door, the monk would unfasten the top end, grab the bottom end and draw it out slowly, knot by knot, hopefully inducing a general rootering out of the plumbing.

Not long ago I read a story about a curious piece of furniture nicknamed the Slant Step that now resides in the Fine Arts Collection of the University of California at Davis. Discovered in the 1960s in a Bay Area junk store, it resembles a small chair, but the seat tilts upward from front to back in a way that makes sitting or standing upon it next to impossible. Artfully made of carved wood, upholstered with a layer of black rubber and then green linoleum, the Slant Step baffled experts for decades. It also inspired many artists who celebrated it as a genius example of eccentric folk art.

Finally, its true purpose was discovered. It was the product of a constipated inventor who used it as a special footstool when he was on the toilet. The angled surface would allow him to hoist his feet and force his knees up toward his chest while seated on the toilet. Coiling his body in this way gave him leverage, apparently, to exert extra pressure on the task at hand.

Wow. A good bowel movement should not be this complicated. Or difficult. It should not require special custom-made furniture. It also should not require whole-body flossing with knotted string. It also should not require hours of massage by strong-handed women (though I'm not saying this is a bad thing).

Nor should a good bowel movement require the regular use of laxatives, lubricating oils, stool softeners, suppositories, colonics, or enemas. Ha! I just said "regular"!

Resorting to extreme measures may be necessary in rare emergency situations. But pushing the panic button too often can mess with your body's natural chemistry and leave you vulnerable to dependency problems. Also, forcing the issue is putting pressure on yourself, and pressure is not conducive to performance in this matter, as I have already stated with great emphasis, offering frightful personal anecdotes to illustrate my point.

A good bowel movement is not a mind-over-matter operation. You can't will yourself to poop any more than you can will yourself to sleep.

No, it must be allowed to happen naturally. The key is to relax. Relax your body by relaxing your mind. Get your brain out of the way of your bowel. Achieve a restful state of thought. It's like classic meditation, but in a slightly different seated position!

I am happy to say I've done much meditation on this matter in recent years, usually with my chin resting on my fist and my elbow resting on my knee, and as a result I can share a number of tips with you:

- **DON'T STRAIN YOURSELF.** You'll break something. Seriously, if you find yourself grunting and groaning on the pot, you're overworking it. And overworking doesn't work.

    Walk away.

- **IT'S A BATHROOM, NOT A LIBRARY.** Don't take reading material into the bathroom. I know this sounds like heresy, coming from an old newspaperman such as myself, but I mean it. Visiting the bathroom with a newspaper in hand, or a book or cell phone or whatever, indicates an assumption on your part that you will be in there for a while. That's not good. It shows you lack confidence. It shows you may not be ready. Trying to go before you are ready is a form of putting pressure on yourself.

    Pressure. Bad!

- **WHEN NATURE CALLS, PICK UP.** Just as you cannot force the urge when it isn't there, you must not fight the urge when it is. Follow nature's plan for your body. If you need to go, by all means, go! Pull off the freeway, or excuse yourself from the meeting, or interrupt your chores, or pause the DVD, or do whatever you need to do to take advantage of this important opportunity.

    I know some people actually resist their first urges. They hoard their load on purpose, in the mistaken hope that waiting until later will produce a greater critical mass with more stupendous results.

    This theory stinks. Straining to delay the event is as bad as, if not worse than, straining to get the event started. Don't try to play control freak with Mother Nature. Go with the flow, so to speak.

- **THE ANSWER, MY FRIEND, IS BLOWING IN THE WIND.** You ask, is
  it also bad to suppress the urge to pass gas? Yes, usually it is.
  Oh, I admit, on occasion it may be acceptable, even advisable,
  to stifle a fart, but it better be for a good reason. You'd better
  be having a quiet tea for two with the Queen of England.
  Or you'd better have just come to a dramatic pause in your
  keynote speech to the shareholders.

    If, on the other hand, you are stoppering farts for no rea-
  son, you are doing yourself a giant disfavor. Alas, once again,
  you are putting pressure on yourself.

    Pressure. Bad!

    Some people worry that "gas leakage" is a waste of the pre-
  cious natural propellant that will be needed later, they hope,
  in the bathroom. On the contrary, farting helps, rather than
  hurts, your chances for on-schedule success. It's a necessary
  part of the process and serves as prod and precursor to the
  main event.

    So, welcome the winds of fortune, my friends. May they fill
  thy sails and speed thee on thy way!

- **A SWARM OF SMALL QUAKES.** Does this ever happen to you:
  You're on the pot, and things have gotten off to a great start
  but then there's a lull in the action. It's frustrating because you
  know you're not done. There's more product to move. You can
  feel it.

    Like most people, I used to sit there, impatiently, waiting
  for Act Two.

    I stopped doing that when I realized that growing impa-
  tient is an application of pressure.

    Pressure. Bad!

    Now, whenever this happens, I play a little trick on my
  system. I get all nonchalant. Have it your way, I say to my
  bowel. I quickly tidy up, leave the bathroom, and attend to

other things. Sure enough, my system usually will say, "Hey, we weren't done yet!"

"OK, have it your way," I'll say again to my bowel. And back we go to the bathroom.

On some days, this little cat-and-mouse game might be repeated several times. I don't mind. I'd rather have several short sessions that get the job done than one marathon session that doesn't. Plus, I feel clever in politely obliging my system to drive the action, not me. It's the way it should be. It's a bodily function, so let the body make the decision.

It's nature's plan. Let nature make the call.

There. I hope some of these tips will be useful to you. And remember the one tip that's the most important of all, because it makes the others less necessary: A plant-strong, fiber-rich diet will make all parts of your body work better.

All parts.

Improve your intake, improve your output. Eat lots of veggies, fruits, greens, and legumes. Good stuff in, easy stuff out.

That's the way to go!

Happy Home Remedies for Digestive Problems

For constipation, a spoonful or two of blackstrap molasses is a time-honored cure. Another classic is eating prunes or raisins or cherries. A teaspoon of castor oil definitely will help lube your pipes. A cup of dandelion tea at night can be helpful. And botanical laxative teas specially formulated with the herb senna are usually very effective for occasional use. These teas are available at health food stores and large markets.

For excessive gas and flatulence, fennel seeds are an ancient remedy, which is why you find them provided as an after-dinner condiment at many Indian restaurants. Fennel can be taken in tea form, too. Other teas to try are ginger, lavender, or peppermint. All are good digestives that can help calm the storm winds in your gut. A couple of spoonfuls of herbal bitters, taken after a meal, can be helpful, too. Bitters typically contain alcohol, so look for them in the liquor aisle. (Don't worry, the tiny amount you'll consume will not compromise your respectability.)

For irritable bowel, raw potatoes or cold boiled potatoes contain resistant starch that creates bulky stool and provides a soothing, protective coating to the inner walls of your gut. Other foods that supply resistant starch are beans and unripe bananas.

CHAPTER EIGHTEEN

Happy Home Remedies

AFTER MY FATHER, HOWARD B. WEEKS, RETIRED FROM ADVENTIST DENOMINA-tional work in the early 1970s, he founded a publishing company, Woodbridge Press, which specialized in books on health and nutrition. Most of these were new titles by new authors, but there was one that dated back more than 200 years. It was *Primitive Remedies*, a reprint edition of a book originally published in 1747 under the title *Primitive Physick*, which in the vernacular of the 1700s meant "Basic Health Care." It was written by John Wesley, the great Protestant reformer and founder of the Methodist Church.

A compilation of natural "cures" for hundreds of common ailments, the book had been enormously popular in its day, before the advent of modern medical science. It was used as a home health manual by generations of families both in Europe and America.

As my father pointed out in his introduction to the Woodbridge Press edition of 1973, many of the homespun remedies found in the book still make perfect sense. For example, here's a "primitive remedy" for constipation, which in the old days was called costiveness: "Take daily, two hours before dinner, a small tea cupful of stewed prunes." That advice is still golden.

On the other hand, some of the old cures seem "quaintly amusing," as Dad put it. One remedy for asthma, for example, was to "live a fort-night on boiled carrots only." A cure for baldness was to rub the head "morning and evening with onions till it is red, and rub it afterwards with honey."

It's no surprise that a centuries-old book of home remedies was known to my father and that he took a fancy to reviving it in print. Our whole family has a special interest in natural medicine that goes back generations. Ellen G. White, though she is most famous for guiding the Adventist church to a vanguard position in the development of modern medical technology, was also very much a believer in nature's healing powers.

In a letter of 1897 to Dr. John Harvey Kellogg, director of the church's famed Battle Creek Sanitarium in Michigan, she wrote, "The Lord has given some simple herbs of the field that at times are beneficial; and if every family were educated in how to use these herbs in case of sickness, much suffering might be prevented, and no doctor need be called. These old-fashioned, simple herbs, used intelligently, would have recovered many sick who have died under drug medication."

Some of my great-great-grandmother's favorite home remedies were well known among her inner circle because she used them often and praised them highly. She believed that catnip tea helps "quiet the nerves," as she put it. For insomnia, she recommended a tea made from the flower of the hop plant. She spoke often of the therapeutic effects of charcoal, pulverized and mixed with water, to be taken orally as a digestive or made into a paste and applied to the skin to treat wounds, inflammation, aches, and pains.

In fact, she extolled the virtues of charcoal at such length in her 1897 letter to Kellogg that she ended by joking that charcoal might seem too good to be true, as humble a substance as it is. "I expect you will laugh at this," she wrote, "but if I could give this remedy some outlandish name that no one knew but myself, it would have greater influence. But the simplest remedies may assist nature, and leave no baleful effects after their use."

In a 1908 letter to John A. Burden, an Adventist administrator at Loma Linda, she told a story about the beneficial use of charcoal that offers a charming autobiographical reference and illustrates the fact that she learned her first lessons in natural medicine as a young girl at home. "My mother has told me that snake bites and the sting of reptiles and poisonous insects could be rendered harmless by the use of charcoal poultices," she wrote.

Ellen G. White was encouraged by her mother to believe in nature's healing power, and she in turn handed down that belief to the generations of her family that followed.

The message still was reverberating loudly and clearly in our family when I came along. Yes, indeed. Ellen G. White's great-granddaughter, Dorothy Mae White Weeks, kept an eagle eye on her first son, little Johnny Weeks. She always was ready to treat any indisposition with any number of unguents and ointments, compounds and compresses, salves and solutions, potions and purgatives, and formulas and fomentations.

Castor oil was a favorite of hers. It's an extract of the castor bean plant and no bottle of it ever lasted long in our house. She would rub it on the painful plantar warts that afflicted the bottoms of my feet. And it worked! She rubbed it on my cuts and bruises and aches and pains. And it worked! She would put drops in my eye to treat infection, and spoonfuls down my throat to treat an upset tummy. And it worked! She even wrestled me to the ground for the occasional castor oil enema, to relieve constipation. And it worked!

I think that at one time or another I was dosed with castor oil everywhere it is possible to be dosed, both inside and outside of my body.

And it worked!

Maybe, as an adult, I should look into keeping a bottle of castor oil in my own house. It's hard to forget how lousy it smells and tastes, though! Ugh.

Meanwhile, I'm going to keep the ball rolling here and pay forward a longtime White/Weeks family tradition by sharing with you a few of the other notable home remedies that have come down to me over the course of generations. As you know, I've included a "Happy Home Remedy" at the end of each chapter of this book so far, but I've saved a couple dozen of my personal favorites for a chapter of their own. Here they are:

Allergies

Irritants in the food we eat and the air we breathe can cause seasonal or chronic allergic reactions that spell misery for millions of us. Congestion, inflammation, swelling, itching—these are just some of the symptoms suffered by the red-eyed, runny-nosed, coughing, wheezing, scratching weary ones who are allergic to pollen, dust, pet dander, certain foods, and other triggers. Home remedies include natural antihistamines such as rooibus (red bush) tea, chamomile tea, and stinging nettle, which is available in both tea and capsule form at health food stores. A time-honored treatment for sinus allergies is to place several drops of eucalyptus oil in boiling water and inhale the steam. An interesting preventive measure against seasonal allergies is to eat a couple of teaspoons of local honey, and chew the beeswax in which it comes, for several days before pollen season starts. The idea is to desensitize your immune system's hostile reaction to local pollens by ingesting the honey made by bees from area pollen.

Bites and Stings

Rub the wound with a cut, raw onion. An application of vinegar will reduce redness and swelling. A paste made by mixing baking soda and water will relieve itchiness. Dabbing with tea tree oil, lavender oil, or peppermint oil can also bring relief. (Not only from the pain but also from the smell of that raw onion that you used first!)

Burns

Aloe vera is nature's miracle cure for minor burns. Always keep a plant in your garden or a windowsill pot. The fresh gel inside the spiky "leaves" of the plant brings cooling, healing relief. Also worth a try: For centuries, Asian cooks have used soy sauce to soothe minor kitchen burns. The condiment is loaded with proteins and antioxidants.

Cramps

Drink a little pickle juice or vinegar. Alternatively, take a spoonful of yellow mustard. Eat a banana. It's full of potassium. The quinine in tonic water is also helpful. Don't look for tonic water in the water aisle. It's in the liquor aisle. It's used in cocktails. I have researched this personally.

Dandruff

Rinse your scalp and hair with vinegar, or tea tree oil diluted with water or shampoo. Or make a hot tea with rosemary, bay leaf, or the herb goldenseal, allow to cool, and then massage the mixture into the scalp.

Fatigue

Here's an old trick known to our ancestors: Cut up an unpeeled potato and soak the pieces in water overnight. Drink the water in the morning to give your body a blast of potassium. It's a tonic for both your nerves and your muscles. If potato water isn't your thing, eat a heaping helping of potassium-rich spinach. It works for Popeye and it'll work for you.

Fever

A steaming hot cup of herbal tea can help you sweat out a fever, especially if it's a tea brewed from one of nature's sweat-inducing plants, such as cayenne pepper, ginger, yarrow, or elderflower. You'll find these teas at the health food store.

Headache

Place an ice pack on the low part of the back of your neck. It draws blood away from the head, which reduces the throbbing. That's what Mom always told me. If you don't have an ice pack, just use anything in your freezer. A bag of frozen peas works just fine. If giving your headache the cold shoulder doesn't work, fight fire with fire and drink a cup of hot herbal tea. Feverfew is a classic remedy for migraine. Other good choices include rosemary, lavender, and peppermint.

Hiccups

I always hold my breath until the hiccups give up and go away. Hiccups are a disruption of your normal breathing pattern, and the cure is to disrupt the disruption. It's like pushing a reset button. Other ways to do it include eating something really sweet (a spoonful of sugar) or sour (vinegar) or sticky (peanut butter) or spicy (hot sauce). Another trick is to breathe into a paper bag, or through a paper towel into a glass.

Indigestion

Mix a ½ teaspoon of baking soda in a small glass of water, drink it down, and prepare to burp your way to relief. Do not overdo the baking soda. Too much of it can cause a volatile reaction in your stomach. You don't want to trade a small problem for a big one.

Nausea

Ginger is nature's champion warrior against queasiness. I am prone to motion sickness, especially in boats on moving water, and I always take a knob of fresh ginger along on such occasions. At the first sign of illness I give the knob a little nibble and, like magic, the nausea disappears. It never fails. Ginger is also available in pill form or as a tea, but I always recommend the fresh stuff.

Nosebleed

A classic home remedy for nosebleed is to hold a cold butter knife against the back of the neck. The sudden chill supposedly triggers a reflex that constricts the blood vessels in the nose. Anything cold will do. It's an old idea. More than two centuries ago, John Wesley's book of *Primitive Remedies* offered these tips for nosebleed: "To cure it, apply to the neck behind, and on each side, a cloth dipped in cold water . . . In a violent case go into a pond or river." Alternatively, you can just do what I do, which is easier. I just pinch my nose, and I pinch hard, until the bleeding stops. It's what I call the hands-on approach to constricting the blood vessels of the nose. It's a lot faster acting than a trip to the river.

Skin Afflictions

It's a pretty safe bet that your grandma and grandpa kept a bottle of witch hazel somewhere handy in the house. The clear extract of the *Hamamelis virginiana* plant, native to North American woodlands, has been used for many centuries, starting with Native Americans, as a natural astringent. It cleanses and soothes skin afflictions of all kinds, including itching, hives, boils, pimples, oily skin, rash, razor burn, sunburn, eczema, and even body odor. For small affected areas, as in the case of a boil or an itchy insect bite, pour witch hazel onto a cotton ball or the corner of a clean washcloth and dab liberally onto the trouble spot. For larger areas, as in the case of a sunburn or rash, use witch hazel even more liberally. Pour some into your hands and slap it on! Ahhh, instant cool relief! You can find witch hazel in drugstores, many large markets, and online.

Snoring

In most cases, snoring hurts your sleep partner more than it hurts you. In worst cases, though, snoring can interfere with your respiration to a dangerous degree, so it's definitely in your own interest to take remedial steps. One old trick is to gargle before bedtime with a homemade mouthwash concocted of a drop or two of peppermint oil in a glass of water. It shrinks the tissues lining your nose and throat, which helps open up your airways.

Toothache

Clove is folk medicine's antidote for the relief of toothache pain. It has natural anesthetic properties. Rub oil of clove on the affected tooth or put a whole clove in your mouth, allow it to moisten and soften, and then use your tongue to hold it against the problem tooth for several minutes. There, feels better, doesn't it?

CHAPTER NINETEEN

Cure for the Common Cold

I WILL BEGIN THIS CHAPTER WITH AN ASTONISHING ANNOUNCEMENT. PLEASE BE seated so that you will not fall to the ground and hurt yourself if you happen to swoon, which is highly likely.

OK, is everyone composed and breathing normally? Here is the announcement:

Common colds are good for us.

Yes, I will give you a moment. Breathe deeply and think pleasant thoughts.

Better?

OK, let me say it again. After years of study and thought on the matter, I am sure that colds are not only good for us, but they are also necessary. They sustain us. Indeed, we could not live without them.

Oh, I know they make us feel miserable. They disrupt our schedules and interfere with our plans. They inconvenience us in every way. We despise them. We consider them an evil.

But we are wrong. We are guilty of a misconception. We judge the common cold unfairly, and we need to cure the way we think about it.

That's what I mean when I title this chapter "Cure for the Common Cold."

OK, OK, calm down. I realize you were expecting something else when you read that title and now you feel swindled. You think I have misled you. But, please, hear me out. Listen to what I have to say, and see if you don't agree with me afterward.

Catching a cold is like buying good insurance. You're paying a little now for a lot of protection later, if and when you need it. Let me explain.

If you are like most people, a cold represents only a minor threat. It's like a little army attacking a big army. The big army is you. Your immune system immediately springs into action when you catch a cold and fights fiercely on your behalf. The battle lasts about a week, and the outcome is almost certain.

Your soldiers win. They vanquish the enemy. They are triumphant. What's more, they are stoked. They are charged up. They feel battle-tested and strong. They are ready for anything that might come next.

And that's good.

You need soldiers like that on your side. You need an army that knows how to fight, because you may well face other, bigger challenges in the future.

Think of those little colds that occasionally come along as the skirmishes that keep your immune system trained and ready for war. You know how we vaccinate ourselves against smallpox and measles by injecting a tiny specimen of the disease into our bloodstream, for the purpose of rallying our antibodies and stimulating them to grow strong against that specific disease? Well, think of the common cold as Mother Nature's little routine vaccination that helps us keep our general defenses up. She offers it periodically, and she doesn't charge us a dime. Thank you, Mother Nature!

My dad must have been almost eighty years old when he told me one day, "You know, it's the most amazing thing, but I've never felt more healthy in my life. It's been years since I even had a cold!"

At the time, I was greatly impressed. I thought, wow, maybe I can look forward to the same thing. I wondered whether it is common for people to enjoy a grace period in late life when they feel fantastic. Immune to colds, even. Golden years indeed!

I hoped my dad would live forever, but he didn't. Oh, he still had several more years to feel better than ever, and never catch so much as a cold, but in his very late eighties, old age and illness managed to get around his defenses and his fantastic run came to an end.

I have to admit, I'm a little superstitious on the subject of colds now. I think I might even start to worry if I enter a long stretch of time when, like my dad, I never catch a cold.

What if it's a trick? What if our immune system gets lulled into a false sense of security? Our soldiers grow old and lazy. They're sluggish. They get rusty. They get out of practice. And, then, when trouble arrives and our health comes under any sort of heavy attack, our soldiers can't muster. They can't rally. They can't even remember what to do.

I don't want to get to that place. I want my soldiers to be up and ready. I don't ever want to stop catching colds.

Colds! Bring them on!

Now, don't get the wrong idea about me as you listen to me rant and rave. I am not getting all smoochy with colds here. I am not saying that we should welcome a cold as a fond friend, or that we should be happy when we get one, or that we should fail to fight against it.

Heck, no.

We should fight colds like crazy. That's the whole point. We catch a cold to fight a cold. Fighting is what keeps us strong.

I grew up in a family that was battle ready and vigilant against any sign of a lurking cold. And, as far back as I can remember, our main weapon was vitamin C.

I have already told you how bemused we all were, in 1970, when Nobel Prize–winning chemist Linus Pauling came out with his best-selling book *Vitamin C and the Common Cold*, in which he argued that megadoses of the vitamin were effective in preventing, treating, and shortening cold symptoms. The book made headlines around the world.

In my family, we all looked at each other and rolled our eyes, as if to say, "Really? Where's this guy been? He's a little late to the party, isn't he?"

It has always been common knowledge in my family that taking vitamin C is the smart thing to do at the first little cough or sniffle. And we don't take just a tablet or two. We take a handful of them—about five of the big 1,000-milligram bombers—and we keep doing it three or four times a day until we are certain that the cold bugs are in full retreat.

That's upward of 20,000 milligrams a day, which is a lot of vitamin C, for sure, but Linus Pauling recommended even more than that. He routinely took 12,000 milligrams a day even when he was healthy, and at the first sign of a cold he jumped it up to 40,000 milligrams. Now, that's a megadose! (The recommended daily allowance for vitamin C is only 60 milligrams a day, by the way.)

Vitamin C is a vital antioxidant that boosts immunity by stimulating production of infection-fighting white blood cells. The medical establishment takes a generally scoffing view of its effectiveness in fighting colds, probably because clinical studies have yielded only mixed results. But those studies typically have been based on vastly smaller dosages of the vitamin than those advocated by Linus Pauling.

And my family.

I know that a healthy respect for vitamin C is an inherited trait for me, going back generations, because I remember always seeing a bottle of vitamin C in Grandpa and Grandma White's house that was just as big as the bottle in our house. And I remember always seeing a big bottle of vitamin C at my Aunt Kay's house. That's Kathryn White Matheson, my mom's sister.

And saying I saw vitamin C at Aunt Kay's house is a little like saying I saw a grain of sand at the beach. It doesn't begin to tell the whole story. Remember, she's the one who founded Full O' Life Natural Foods Market and Restaurant in Burbank, one of Southern California's first and best health food stores, which contains a whole department devoted to natural remedies, including vitamin C and many, many others.

Some time ago, I joined a nice little crowd of the extended family for dinner at Kay's house. There were four generations of us on hand. The meal was excellent, and we all were much contented and ready for conversation when it was done.

I had already begun work on this book, and I was looking ahead to the chapter on cold remedies, which you are reading now, so I put the question to every person at the dinner table: "What do you do when you feel a cold coming on?"

It goes without saying that vitamin C was prominently mentioned, but many other curatives made the list, too. I took good notes, so here goes:

- **VITAMINS AND MINERALS:** Zinc, vitamin C, vitamin D, and vitamin E.
- **BOTANICALS:** Astragalus, echinacea, elderberry, garlic, ginger, goldenseal, horehound, horseradish, licorice, olive leaf, pennyroyal, red raspberry leaf, slippery elm, thyme, and wild Mediterranean oregano oil. Most are available in several forms, including fresh, pill, tincture, and tea.
- **COMMERCIAL HOMEOPATHIC FORMULATIONS:** Hyland's #4 Ferrum Phosphoricum (more info: hylands.com) and Boiron Oscillococcinum (more info: oscillo.com).

In addition to contributing to this list, a number of the people present at Aunt Kay's dinner table that day had some good stories to tell.

It was remembered, for example, that Ellen G. White had a very interesting cold remedy. She would drink a hot cup of sweat-producing cayenne pepper tea. Now, she never mentioned this in her public writings. In fact, her official position on hot peppers was to caution against them because of their stimulant effects, which she compared to the effects produced by caffeine and nicotine. But I did a little follow-up research, after my dinner at Aunt Kay's house, and I discovered that she did mention the cayenne pepper cold remedy on several occasions in her private correspondence.

For example, in a letter of August 21, 1877, to her son James Edson White, she tells how she prescribed it for her husband James: "Your father had a very ill turn yesterday which greatly alarmed us all . . . In the morning he said he felt rather bad. I prepared a cup of weak red pepper tea."

Years later, while traveling on August 27, 1905, she wrote to C. C. Crisler, head of the secretarial staff at Elmshaven, her home in St. Helena, California: "I had an ill turn that night. The wind came up while we were searching for a place to rest. I think I took cold. I was in such severe pain I called for cayenne pepper and obtained some relief."

Here's another story told around Aunt Kay's dinner table that day not so very long ago. I remember it well, because I'm the one who told it. Both my mother and my first mother-in-law used to talk about eating a whole raw onion as a sure cure for a cold. To be honest, I never saw either one of them do it, but I was impressed enough to try it myself. I think it works.

It's not easy, believe me. It takes sheer bravery, and maybe a little treachery.

To eat a raw onion like an apple, right out of your hand, you better find a mighty sweet one. Another trick is to cut it up and eat it in a sandwich that is loaded with other stuff, including tomato, pickles, and strong greens like parsley or radish sprouts, all served between slices of hearty flavorful bread such as rye or pumpernickel. By the way, one of Ernest Hemingway's favorite sandwiches was raw onion and peanut butter on crusty white bread. He mentions it in his novel *Islands in the Stream*, where he calls it "one of the highest points in the sandwich-maker's art. We call it the Mount Everest Special. For Commanders Only."

I have to confess, my usual method of eating a raw onion is to cheat a little bit. I chop the onion, then microwave it in a bowl for a minute or two to blunt its pungency, then drizzle it with maple or agave syrup, and eat it with a spoon. I know, I know. Ernest Hemingway would be ashamed.

Finally, here's a story from Aunt Kay's dinner table that was told by Aunt Kay herself. She remembered that her grandmother, Ethel May White, the wife of Ellen G. White's son Willie, would fight a cold by drinking a potion of fresh grape juice with raw egg yolk whipped into it.

Yikes. I suppose that's a rich brew of antioxidant vitamin C and protein, but I'm not enticed by that combination of flavors! Besides, I'm not eating a lot of animal protein these days, and that includes eggs.

Speaking of animal protein from chickens, I have to report that chicken soup also received a lot of notice around Aunt Kay's dinner table that day. To be honest, I don't eat chicken soup, and I debated whether to even mention it here. On the other hand, it's rather difficult to ignore chicken soup's stature as a classic cold remedy. After some thought, and a good deal of experimentation, I believe I have solved the dilemma in an inventive way. Read on.

A Happy Home Remedy for the Common Cold

Next time you feel under the weather, enjoy a steaming hot bowl of chicken soup . . . without the chicken.

Please, hear me out.

Chicken soup has a reputation as a cold fighter that dates back to antiquity. The Judaic philosopher and physician Moses Maimonides (1135–1204) prescribed it in medieval times, which may help explain how chicken soup ultimately earned the nickname "Jewish penicillin." In modern times, science has lent credence to the folklore surrounding chicken soup. Clinical studies have demonstrated that it has amino acids and proteins that help the body fight inflammation, congestion, and bacterial infection. That's good news.

And here's even better news. It's not the chicken that works the magic in chicken soup. It's the compounds found in the chicken that do the trick, and all those compounds can be found readily in plant foods.

That's right, it's not necessary for chickens to die in order for us to live through the discomforts of a cold. And that's a break for us as well as the chickens. We can gain all the healthful benefits of chicken soup without the unhealthful risks of eating dead carcass meat.

The cysteine in chicken that helps loosen congestion in our body is available in high-protein plant foods such as beans. Beans also contain zinc, a proven immunity booster. The cytokines in chicken that boost our body's immune response to inflammation are abundant in dark, leafy greens. The garlic and onion found in most chicken soups are rich in the natural germ killers alliin and allicin that help our bodies fight bacterial infection.

Here's my own recipe for chicken soup without the chicken. It has beans, leafy greens and other vegetables, and plenty of garlic and onion. Also, I like to "soup it up" with a little hot pepper for extra sinus-clearing congestion relief, plus the herb thyme for cough relief. Believe me, this is better than chicken soup! And it's much faster acting, too, because you can make it in about a half hour instead of the four hours that many chicken soup recipes require.

VEGAN PENICILLIN
(OR, CHICKEN SOUP WITHOUT THE CHICKEN)

Serves 8–10

2 onions, chopped

2 tablespoons olive oil

2 (15-ounce) cans white beans, rinsed and drained

8 cloves garlic, minced

2 carrots, chopped

3 celery stalks, chopped

1 zucchini, chopped

1 potato, peeled and chopped

12 cups water

1 teaspoon ground dried rosemary

1 teaspoon ground dried thyme

1 teaspoon ground dried cayenne pepper

2 dried bay leaves

2 cups uncooked fettuccine pasta, broken into 2-inch pieces

3 cups chopped fresh kale or baby spinach

Kosher salt, black pepper, and crushed red pepper flakes to taste

1. In a deep soup pot over medium heat, stir the chopped onions in the olive oil for 3 minutes.
2. Add the beans, garlic, and fresh vegetables, stir to mix, then add the water, rosemary, thyme, cayenne pepper, and bay leaves. Bring to a boil, then reduce the heat and simmer for 20 minutes.
3. Add the pasta and continue to simmer for 10 minutes.
4. Remove the bay leaves, add the kale or spinach, and continue to simmer for 5 minutes, until the greens are wilted.
5. Remove from the heat and add the salt, pepper, and pepper flakes to taste.

CHAPTER TWENTY

Good Health—
Don't Myth Out

THROUGHOUT HISTORY, PEOPLE HAVE BEEN SUCKERS FOR ANY NEW THING THAT is billed as a cure-all for the maladies that plague us. Everyone wants to live longer and have better health. It's worth everything. And people have always been willing to pay anything.

We all have heard the crazy stories of old times, when hucksters and swindlers roamed the land, making fools of people by selling them strange potions and outlandish contraptions in exchange for exorbitant amounts of money. We shake our heads when we hear such anecdotes of long ago. How gullible those poor people must have been! What a shame, we think.

But you know what's even sadder?

It's much worse now.

There are still armies of magic-formula and miracle-machine sellers, but they have much more power now, and much more sway over people's minds and money than ever before.

In the old days, con artists were itinerants, moving from town to town in creaky mule-drawn wagons, attracting small crowds at a time. Today's grifters use the internet, they use television, and they use many other forms of multimedia communication, which means they have worldwide outreach that enables them to rob millions of people at once, simultaneously, in mere seconds of time.

Today's version of the old snake-oil merchants do not come to our towns and set up tents in a field. No, they reach right into our homes, embracing us individually and collectively on our electronic devices, and they cast their spells, just like their counterparts of centuries past. But today's spells are more dangerous because they have today's state-of-the-art production values. There are pop-up ads all over the internet that link us to flashy websites full of bells and whistles. There are legions of telemarketers who ring us up wherever we happen to be. There are Hollywood-style infomercials on TV with celebrity guests, studio audiences, and applause signs. And operators standing by to take our calls! And special offers if we call right away!

It's harder than ever to separate fact from fiction in this new world of hyper-hucksterism.

I had to laugh the other day when I happened to catch the last part of one TV show where a doctor was discussing the potential risks of taking probiotics (live bacteria used as a dietary supplement), immediately followed by another show in which probiotics were extolled with much fervor as the key to eternal life!

In the old days, misinformation thrived because news traveled so slowly. Today, it flourishes because news travels so quickly, and there is such a constant overload of it, loud and unfiltered, beating us down, battering our defenses, seemingly every waking second of our lives.

One thing hasn't changed. The nutrition and fitness myths of today are exactly like the nutrition and fitness myths of yesterday in that they are obstacles that must be overcome by anyone who chooses to seek the truth about better health.

Tomatoes were considered to be poisonous when they first arrived in Europe in the 1500s on the ships of explorers returning from South America. The Europeans admired their appearance, and used them as decorative objects, much as we use holly berries today, but they wouldn't dare eat them. In a 1597 botanical reference work titled *Herball, or*

Generall Historie of Plantes, author John Gerard warned that the tomato is a toxic plant of "ranke and stinking savour."

It literally took centuries for word to spread, first from southern Europe to northern Europe in the 1600s, and then from northern Europe to North America in the late 1700s and early 1800s, that, hey, people are eating these things and they don't kill you! In fact, they taste good!

Today, of course, in our modern world of instant mass communication, the big tomato controversy would be solved right away, right?

Well, maybe not.

Yes, it's now easy for all of us to talk together, all at once, but for some reason that doesn't seem to translate into making our arguments easier to resolve.

If anything, we get more conflicting messages than ever.

Eggs are good for us. No, eggs are bad.

Chocolate is a vice. No, it's a virtue.

Margarine is better than butter. No, butter is better than margarine.

Coconut oil is evil. No, it's righteous.

Don't drink wine. Wait, drink wine.

Running is better than walking. Wait, walking is better.

(Where do I stand on these important questions? I don't eat eggs, butter, or margarine. I love dark chocolate, but not milk chocolate. I always choose coconut oil that is labeled both "virgin" and "organic." I love wine. Walking makes me feel good. Running hurts.)

I am alternately annoyed and amused by the flip-flopping that takes place in the health and fitness marketplace. How to account for it? First, there's plenty of shady research. To use a farcical example, a nutrition study funded by the Dirt Sandwich Council is sure to render a report that dirt sandwiches are very, very healthful to eat.

Even the squeaky-clean research takes place under extreme pressure because there is competition for funding and attention and, thus, clear motive to report possibly newsworthy findings as they occur, no matter how preliminary or even premature those findings might prove to be.

And the news media, of course, exists in a competitive environment, too, so there is no "sitting on the story," waiting patiently for years, even decades, before a study's final conclusions are presented. No, each development is rushed into print as it is announced, never minding the fact that the final results, years away, may be quite contrary to the early indications that were first reported.

We call this the Information Age, but unfortunately there seems to be as much Bad Information as Good Information. The kind of old-fashioned fact-checked news that used to appear in reliable newspapers and news magazines seems to be going out of fashion as people now look for their news on the internet, where liars and idiots outnumber experts a million to one.

Crooks and crackpots, scammers and scoundrels have been with us always, of course, but they possess a much longer reach now, so it's more difficult than ever to sort out the sense from the nonsense. Who knows? We may start hearing any day from some blogger or another that tomatoes are deadly poisonous!

I swear, I could write a whole book about nutrition and fitness myths, and there would be plenty of swearing in it, I guarantee. Misconceptions about food and fitness represent a real threat, I feel, and the warnings against them should be strong enough to get people's attention.

Maybe I'll write that book next. For now, I'll just mention a few of the real doozies that bug me the most. Every time I hear them, I wonder whether to laugh or cry. Sometimes I do both.

Myth: Exercise Should Hurt

The adage "No Pain, No Gain" is not only wrong but also dangerous. Don't listen to the gym rats. Take your advice from sensible fitness experts. Here's a statement from Loma Linda University Health, the umbrella organization that manages all of LLU's programs and services (more info: lomalindauniversityhealth.org): "You don't need to feel pain to have a good workout. In fact, pushing yourself too hard during exercise can lead to injury, including sprains and fractures."

The idea is to improve your body, not damage it. Steer clear of routines that punish. Avoid workout equipment that traumatizes. Remember that some of the most effective exercises are the simplest—including, of course, what I call the world's best exercise: walking!

Myth: Feed a Cold, Starve a Fever

Proper nutrition and hydration are essential when you are healthy, and urgently essential when you are ill. You must replenish the nutrients and fluids that illness depletes from your body. Eat food and drink plenty of fluids whenever you are sick—with or without fever.

Myth: Artificial Sweeteners Are an Ideal Alternative to Sugar

Chemical sweeteners became widely used starting in the 1950s, which means we've been drinking diet sodas and eating sugar-free foods for about sixty years. So, why aren't we skinny yet? In fact, why have we gotten fatter with each decade since then? There are many studies that raise serious questions about artificial sweeteners. Do they actually boost our craving for sweets, because they don't naturally fulfill that craving the way sugar does? Do they confuse the brain's natural ability to measure food intake, causing the brain to signal the body that it needs more to eat? A 2004 study at Purdue University found that laboratory animals that swigged an artificially sweetened liquid were more likely to gain weight than those who drank a naturally sweetened liquid. That's because the first group did a lot of binge eating of high-calorie foods while the second group ate more moderately.

And, honestly, we don't need to rely on laboratory animal studies to reach this conclusion, do we? We all see this identical behavior with our own eyes in the human population, right? Visit any fast food restaurant and watch people ordering double bacon cheeseburgers and greasy french fries . . . and a diet drink! Poor confused people. As for myself, I avoid artificial sweeteners and take it easy with sugar, too. That way, I don't have to worry about either one of them.

Myth: Canned or Frozen Fruits and Vegetables Are a Poor Alternative to Fresh Produce

Who started this lie? I'll bet it was someone who didn't like fruits and vegetables and looked for any excuse to avoid eating them. The fact is, fruits and vegetables that are harvested and then immediately flash frozen or sealed in cans or bottles may have more of their vital nutrients intact than "fresh" produce that has spent days or even weeks of travel time in trucks and railroad cars. To be sure, there's nothing better than fresh produce that is truly fresh—straight from the farm to your table. But if you didn't make it to the farmers' market last weekend, and the produce at your market is looking a little ragged, there is nothing wrong with channeling your inner Green Giant and mixing a fine succotash of canned or frozen lima beans, corn, peppers, onions, and stewed tomatoes. There are no excuses. Eat your fruits and veggies!

Myth: Chile Peppers Are Hard on Your Stomach

Nonsense. Have I already told you the story of how I used to buy antacids in the jumbo-size bottles? How I used to carry antacids around in my shirt pockets? How I used to scarf antacids all the time? Then, in the 1980s, I became a chile head after a glorious week of restaurant dining in Santa Fe, New Mexico, where every dish on every plate is loaded with jalapeños, pasillas, poblanos, serranos, habaneros, guajillos, and other peppers. The food not only tasted awesome, but it also made me feel awesome, all day long and all night long. I've loved spicy food ever since and, what's more, I rarely need to use antacids anymore.

So, friends, it is with all the enthusiasm of a true believer that I report to you that clinical study after clinical study has demonstrated that hot peppers are good for you, not bad for you. Capsaicin, the chemical compound that gives hot peppers their heat, actually soothes and protects your stomach and digestive system, because it inhibits the secretion of stomach acid. As reported in the *New England Journal of Medicine* (March 2002), researchers in one study were so impressed by the palliative effect of hot peppers on indigestion that they suggested that capsaicin might be considered a primary medical therapy for the condition. Let's put that a different way: Hot chile peppers don't cause heartburn, they cure it!

Capsaicin has already been used for years as the active ingredient in many pain-relief ointments applied to the skin. Turns out, capsaicin is also good for what ails us when applied internally, via chile peppers! In fact, ongoing research indicates that capsaicin may hold promise as a natural wonder drug that helps combat even the most serious diseases, including arthritis, hypertension, diabetes, even cancer. An international longevity study reported in the August 2015 edition of the *British Medical Journal* found that eating spicy hot foods several times a week may add years to our lives because of capsaicin's remarkable anti-inflammatory properties.

Another study, at Nottingham University in England, found that capsaicin actually kills cancer cells without harming surrounding healthy cells. Lead researcher Dr. Timothy Bates told the BBC, "We believe that we have in effect discovered a fundamental 'Achilles heel' for all cancer."

Moral of the story: Don't hesitate to turn up the heat in what you eat!

Myth: A Meat Diet Is Necessary for Complete Nutrition

What a crock. The complete opposite is true. In fact, it is necessary to limit or ideally remove meat from your diet in order to optimize your nutrition, your health, and your life expectancy. The "meat is necessary" myth is the biggest, worst health lie of all, because it harms the most people. It dooms countless millions of them to disease, disability, and early death. It stands in the way of countless millions of them who could make better choices if they knew the truth.

Here's the truth:

You don't need meat for protein. A healthy diet that includes lots of vegetables, beans, grains, and nuts will deliver all the protein your body needs.

You don't need red meat for iron. In fact, green vegetables and beans are better than red meat because they deliver iron in a form that is more efficiently absorbed by the human body.

You don't need fish for omega-3 fatty acids. Soybeans, walnuts, flax-seeds, dark leafy greens, and other plants offer a better source. Unlike fish, which contains unhealthy saturated fats as well as healthy omega-3 fats, plants deliver only the good fat. Why take the good with the bad, when you can have the good *without* the bad?

You don't need dairy products for calcium. In fact, vegetables build better bones than milk and eggs do. Dark leafy greens are not only rich in calcium, but they also deliver bone-fortifying vitamins K and D, which dairy products don't. Vitamin D often is inserted into dairy milk, as an additive, but it comes naturally in collard greens, kale, bok choy, and other greens. Nuts, oats, and potatoes deliver calcium plus bone-building magnesium, which dairy products don't. Nut, soy, and rice milks are excellent alternatives to cow milk, plus they are lactose-free, which solves the allergy problem for people who are lactose-intolerant.

Health myths like these won't go away. That's why we need to remain on our guard against them. At best, they are a distraction. At worst, they are a deadly threat.

In all cases, they complicate our quest for a better life. Once we move around them, and beyond them, we find that the truth is not far in the distance.

In fact, the truth is right in front of us.

Ellen G. White was telling the truth 150 years ago, and modern science is proving it today. The meaty diet favored in much of the Western world is toxic to humans. It promotes obesity and disease. Most meat eaters will die poisoned by the food that they eat.

There is a solution. Food can be the hero instead of the villain in our lives. A plant-based whole foods diet of fresh fruits, vegetables, leafy greens, whole grains, nuts, seeds, and legumes keeps our bodies clean and lean, and protects us from disease. We can live better, live stronger, live longer.

Ready to try it yourself?

It won't cost you an extra penny. In fact, you'll start saving all that money you used to spend on crazy diets and bogus miracle drugs and scary exercise machines.

Your grocery bill will go down. So will your cholesterol, your blood sugar, your blood pressure, your body fat, your weight, and your stress level.

It's the best deal there is, and you can take advantage of it any time you like.

You can start right now.

Happy Home Remedies for Meat Dependence

Longtime vegetarians and vegans are a happy bunch, but brand-new vegetarians and vegans are even happier because they also are amazed! They are amazed at how good their food tastes and how good they feel. They are amazed they waited so long to make the switch.

Hey, it's OK to be a little nervous before making a big change. Here's a short list of tips that might help out:

- **MAKE IT EASY.** Don't try to quit cold turkey, so to speak, unless that works for you. It's OK to take it in stages. Start with Meatless Monday, then expand it to Meatless Monday and Thursday. Gradually add more days. Or, instead of taking a calendar approach, take a category approach. First, cut red meat from your diet. Next, cut white meat. Then fish. Then dairy, if you're going all the way.
- **MAKE IT FUN.** Spread the news, tell all your friends, gain supporters. Brag a lot. Take lots of "before" selfies so you can compare them later with the "after"

selfies that will show you looking slimmer and healthier. Keep bragging. Start discovering all the great vegetarian restaurants in town and ethnic restaurants that offer delicious meatless dishes. Become an expert. Keep bragging. Become a collector of great vegetarian recipes. Start creating your own. Start throwing vegetarian parties. Keep bragging.

- **MAKE IT REAL.** Combine your new diet with new goals, such as losing weight or running a marathon or starting a new job. Or a new romance. It's great when you get multiple motivating factors working together for you.

- **MAKE IT REASONABLE.** If you yield to temptation and eat a hot dog at the ballpark on the delirious day your team wins the World Series, don't condemn yourself to damnation. Forgive yourself this one time, and go forth. Get back on track. It's OK to falter, as long as you don't fail. Oh, and by the way, most Major League ballparks now offer veggie dogs, veggie burgers, or other vegetarian food items, so check that out next time!

- **MAKE IT SUSTAINABLE.** Vegetarians and vegans still must make smart food choices and eat well-balanced, complete meals. Careless vegetarians and vegans can eat very poorly, and fare very badly. Noodles are meat-free, but a carbo-loading human who eats nothing but noodles is bound to get fatter and sicker, not slimmer and healthier. French fries are vegan. Sugar is vegan. But if your diet mainly consists of french fries and sugar, you will not flourish. No, what you want to eat, every day, for the rest of your longer, better life, is a plant-based whole foods diet that is multidimensional and complete, with a rich array of vegetables, leafy greens, beans, fruits, nuts, and grains. It's the world's best diet!

- **MAKE IT EXCITING.** Your new diet is a reward, not a punishment. It's a cause for celebration. Think about the new, wonderful things you're eating, not the old, nasty stuff you don't eat anymore. Keep track of the weight you lose, marvel at the new energy you feel. Log the extra number of miles you now can walk or run. Give yourself a treat as you reach new milestones: that first meat-free week, that first meat-free month, that first meat-free year.

Break out the champagne!

It's vegan.

Cheers!

CHAPTER TWENTY-ONE

John's Omnipotent Recipes

OK, THAT'S ENOUGH TALK. LET'S EAT!

The best way to embrace and celebrate a plant-based whole foods diet is to put good food on the table. So let's do that. Here are forty-two special recipes to get us started. I call them "omnipotent" because, in most cases, they each offer a complete nutrition profile, with ingredients that represent the entire range of essential food groups: proteins, healthy carbohydrates, fruits, and vegetables. Each one of these four components, by itself, is a potent source of nutritional goodness. Together, in one dish, they are omnipotent!

Many of these recipes come from my own family, written by hand on bits of paper that in some cases are more than a hundred years old. There are recipes from my mother, my grandmother, and even my great-great-grandmother. Learn how to make Ellen G. White's favorite breakfast dish, her favorite noodle dish, her favorite salad, and her favorite dessert. These exclusive family recipes appear here in print for the first time anywhere.

BREAKFAST

THE REAL DEAL OATMEAL

Serves 4

Scottish oatmeal is made the ancient way, by stone grinding whole oat groats into a coarse meal (hence the name *oatmeal*). The process yields a whole-grain product with its germ, oil, and fiber intact. You'll find Scottish oatmeal in the cereal aisle at many large markets, most health food stores, and online.

> 3 cups water
> Dash of salt
> 1 cup Scottish oatmeal
> 2 bananas, peeled and sliced
> ½ cup raw or roasted cashews
> ½ cup blueberries
> ¼ cup roasted unsalted pumpkin seeds (pepitas)
> Maple syrup, for drizzling (optional)

1. Bring the water and salt to a boil in a saucepan over medium-high heat. Add the oatmeal, reduce the heat to low, cover, and cook for 10 minutes, stirring occasionally. Remove from the heat and let stand for 2 minutes.
2. Mix in the bananas and cashews.
3. Divide among four serving bowls. Sprinkle each with blueberries and pumpkin seeds and drizzle with maple syrup, if desired.

Food groups: protein (cashews), carbohydrate (oatmeal), fruit (blueberries, bananas), vegetable (pumpkin seeds)

PEANUT-PINEAPPLE RICE

Serves 4-6

If I see cooked rice in front of me, my first instinct is to stick a big spoon of peanut butter in it and stir it up. I'll even intervene if someone at my table at an Asian restaurant suggests leaving behind what's left of the ubiquitous bowl of steamed or fried rice.

"No, I'll take it home and eat it tomorrow with peanut butter," I will say.

I love the flavor combination of peanut and rice. Turns out, it's hereditary. My parents liked it, my grandfather liked it, and both he and his sister Grace would recount how their own grandmother, Ellen G. White, was fond of it. Just a simple bowl of hot rice with peanut butter stirred into it.

Here's a recipe that's a bit fancier than that, but it honors those flavors.

4 cups water, divided
2 cups uncooked brown rice
1 tablespoon vegetable oil
2 scallions, chopped
1 tablespoon soy sauce
2 tablespoons tomato paste
¼ cup creamy peanut butter
2 cups fresh pineapple chunks
½ cup chopped fresh cilantro

1. Bring 3 cups of the water to a boil in a saucepan, add the rice, stir, cover, reduce the heat to low, and cook for about 30 minutes, or until all the water is absorbed. Remove from the heat and let rest for 10 minutes, covered, then fluff with a fork.
2. Heat the oil in a small saucepan, add the onions, and stir for 1 minute. Add the soy sauce, tomato paste, and the remaining 1 cup of water and stir to blend.
3. Add the peanut butter and stir for 1 minute until a smooth sauce is formed.
4. Add the pineapple chunks to the cooked rice and stir to combine.
5. Place the rice in a serving bowl and pour the peanut sauce over the top. Sprinkle with the chopped cilantro.

Food groups: *protein (peanut butter), carbohydrate (brown rice), fruit (pineapple, tomato paste), vegetable (scallion, cilantro)*

BUCKWHEAT GRIDDLE CAKES WITH CRUSHED STRAWBERRIES

Serves 4-8 (makes 8 griddle cakes)

After you've feasted on these, you'll never look at plain pancakes in quite the same way. In fact, you probably won't bother looking at plain pancakes at all.

2 cups whole-grain buckwheat flour
2 teaspoons baking powder
2 cups unsweetened almond milk
¼ cup unsweetened applesauce
24 fresh strawberries, crushed
¼ cup toasted slivered almonds (see Note)
1 cup fresh mint leaves

1. In mixing bowl, whisk the flour and baking powder. Add the almond milk and applesauce and stir to combine. Allow the batter to rest for 10 minutes.

2. Coat a frying pan with cooking spray and heat over medium heat. For each griddle cake, pour ¼ cup batter into the pan and cook until the edges are firm and bubbles appear on the surface (2–3 minutes), then flip and cook until done (about 2 minutes). Repeat for each additional griddle cake.

3. To serve, spoon crushed strawberries over each griddle cake, sprinkle with toasted almond slivers, and garnish with mint leaves.

Food groups: *protein (almonds), carbohydrate (buckwheat flour), fruit (applesauce, strawberries), vegetable (mint)*

NOTE: To toast almonds or any other nuts or seeds, stir constantly in a dry pan over medium heat until they just start to brown. Remove the pan immediately from the heat and continue to stir constantly for 1 minute, then pour into a shallow dish to cool.

THE SUPER BOWL

Serves 1

I always keep lots of fresh fruit and greens and nuts in the kitchen, and this recipe is one of the reasons why. It's so easy to put together, so beautiful to look at, and so good to eat. It's one of my favorite breakfasts.

¼ cup raw old-fashioned (rolled) oats
½ cup fresh strawberries, cut into quarters
1 small apple, unpeeled, chopped
1 small juicy orange, peeled and sectioned

1 small banana, peeled and cut into thick slices
½ cup fresh cilantro leaves, cut into strips
2 seedless dates, chopped
2 tablespoons chopped raw walnuts
1 tablespoon ground flaxseed meal
1 tablespoon unsweetened coconut flakes

1. Combine the oats, strawberries, chopped apple, and orange segments with all their juice, and mix well.
2. Mix in the banana slices, cilantro leaves, dates, and nuts.
3. Sprinkle with the flaxseed meal and coconut flakes and serve.

Food groups: protein (walnuts, flaxseed), carbohydrate (oats), fruit (orange, apple, banana, strawberries, dates, coconut), vegetable (cilantro)

ELLEN G. WHITE'S FAVORITE BREAKFAST: COOKED WHEAT BERRIES WITH FRUIT AND NUTS

Serves 4–6

My great-great-grandmother loved hot whole-grain cereal served in a bowl with fresh cream. Wheat, oats, rice, millet, cornmeal—all varieties of grain were to her liking. She also insisted on several kinds of fresh fruit with the morning meal. And nuts. She was crazy about nuts. She bought almonds by the hundred-pound bag!

Here's her original recipe for a breakfast dish for four to six people that combines wheat berries, fresh fruits, and almonds. Wheat berries are entire wheat kernels with the bran, germ, and endosperm intact. They are readily available at health food stores and online.

My great-great-grandmother had her wheat berries cooked the old-fashioned way, brought to a boil in a pot of water, and then left to soak in the tightly covered hot water overnight. They would be ready to eat in the morning. But the same result can be achieved in much less time by bringing the wheat berries to a boil, lowering the heat, and cooking for about an hour until tender.

2 cups whole wheat berries
6 cups water

2 bananas, peeled and sliced
1 cup dates, pitted and chopped
½ cup raisins
¼ cup slivered almonds
Soy or almond milk (optional)

1. Combine wheat berries and water in a pot and bring to a boil over medium-high heat. Reduce the heat to low and cook, covered, for 50–60 minutes, until tender.
2. Drain and divide the cooked wheat berries among 4–6 serving bowls. Top each with banana slices, dates, raisins, and almonds.
3. Add a splash of soy milk, if desired.

Food groups: *protein (almonds), carbohydrate (wheat berries), fruit (bananas, dates, raisins), vegetable (soy milk)*

....

TIP: Ellen G. White liked to pour fresh dairy cream over her cereal, but it's easy to turn this dish vegan by substituting soy or almond milk.

....

MUSH 'N' SHROOMS

Serves 4–6

Making polenta is easy. It's basically just cornmeal mush. Stir-frying some mushrooms is easy, too. Now, what happens when you combine polenta and stir-fried mushrooms? Wow, it's easily one of the best breakfast dishes you'll ever eat. You might start making it for lunch and dinner, too!

FOR THE POLENTA:
3 cups soy milk
1 cup whole-grain cornmeal
Pinch of salt
3 tablespoons dairy-free butter spread (see Note)

FOR THE MUSHROOMS:
¼ cup extra virgin olive oil
3 tablespoons dairy-free butter spread
1 teaspoon ground sage
1 teaspoon ground rosemary

1 teaspoon garlic powder

1 pound mixed fresh mushrooms (such as cremini, portobello, shiitake, porcini, or chanterelle), coarsely chopped

¼ cup vegetable broth or water

1 tablespoon sherry vinegar

¼ teaspoon black pepper

TO MAKE THE POLENTA:

1. In a medium-size pan, bring the soy milk to a simmer over medium heat.
2. Slowly stir in the cornmeal, add the salt, and reduce the heat to low. Cook, stirring often to prevent sticking, for 30–40 minutes, until the polenta is creamy and tender.
3. Remove from the heat, stir in the dairy-free butter spread, and set aside for a few minutes to thicken.

TO MAKE THE MUSHROOMS:

1. Combine the olive oil, dairy-free butter spread, sage, rosemary, and garlic powder in a large skillet and stir over medium heat until the butter spread is melted and the mixture is smooth.
2. Add the mushrooms, stir to coat, increase the heat to high, and cook until the mushrooms begin to brown, 3–4 minutes.
3. Add the vegetable broth, stir well, and then remove from the heat.
4. Add the vinegar, stir well, and sprinkle with the black pepper.

TO SERVE:

1. Transfer the prepared polenta to a serving dish and top with the mushrooms.

Food groups: *protein (soy milk), carbohydrate (polenta), vegetable (mushrooms)*

- -

NOTE: Dairy-free butter spread is available in the dairy aisle of many large markets and health food stores.

- -

MONKEY-BUNNY CAKE

Serves 6-8

The monkey was in the kitchen getting ready to make monkey bread with bananas when all of a sudden the bunny showed up and offered to help. Naturally, the bunny had brought carrots and wanted to add them to the mix. The result was Monkey-Bunny Cake!

What, you've never heard this story? Well, it's not surprising, because I just made it up. I made up this recipe, too. It's really good. It goes great with your morning coffee.

2 cups whole-grain pastry flour
2 teaspoons baking soda
½ teaspoon salt
1 cup sugar
¼ cup vegetable oil
3 ripe bananas, mashed
1 carrot, grated
¼ cup water
1 teaspoon vanilla extract
½ cup chopped walnuts
Frozen peaches, slightly thawed (optional)

1. Preheat the oven to 350 degrees. Coat a 9-inch square cake pan or baking dish with cooking spray.
2. Combine the flour, baking soda, and salt in a bowl and stir to blend.
3. In a separate bowl, combine the sugar and oil. Add the mashed bananas and grated carrot and mix thoroughly. Add the water and vanilla and mix thoroughly.
4. Add the flour mixture and chopped walnuts and mix thoroughly.
5. Spread into the prepared pan and bake for 40–50 minutes, until lightly browned on top.
6. Let the bread cool in the pan, then turn out onto a cooling rack to cool completely. Serve with slightly thawed frozen peaches, if desired. Yummy!

Food groups: *protein (walnuts), carbohydrate (flour), fruit (bananas), vegetable (carrot)*

LUNCH

PEANUT BUTTER POWER SANDWICH

Serves 1

This takes almost no time to make. It takes a little longer to eat, though, because you'll linger over each peanut-buttery bite with a big smile on your face.

2-3 tablespoons unsalted peanut butter (or any nut butter)
2 slices sturdy whole-grain bread, lightly toasted
1-2 tablespoons chopped red onion
1-2 tablespoons raisins
1 small banana, thickly sliced
1 handful fresh baby spinach leaves

1. Spread the peanut butter on both slices of bread.
2. On one of the slices, sprinkle the chopped onion and raisins. Arrange the banana slices on top and cover with the spinach leaves.
3. Press the other slice of bread into place to complete the sandwich. Slice into halves or quarters, if desired.

Food groups: *protein (peanut butter, spinach), carbohydrate (bread), fruit (raisins, banana), vegetable (onion, spinach)*

GRILLED PORTOBELLO MUSHROOM BURGERS

Serves 4

The plant world takes on the animal world in the battle of the burgers. And the plant world wins!

¼ cup balsamic vinegar
2 tablespoons olive oil
1 teaspoon dried basil
1 teaspoon dried oregano
4 large fresh portobello mushrooms, rinsed, with stems and membranes removed

1 (15-ounce) can kidney beans, rinsed and drained

2 tablespoons vegan steak sauce (such as A1 brand)

4 whole-grain wheat hamburger buns

1 red onion, sliced

2 ripe tomatoes, sliced

Handful of fresh lettuce (any variety)

1. Preheat a grill to medium-high or preheat the oven to 400 degrees.
2. Combine the vinegar, oil, basil, and oregano in a large bowl and whisk until thoroughly blended. Add the mushrooms and turn to coat on all sides.
3. Grill for 10 minutes, turning after 5 minutes, or bake for 20 minutes, turning after 10 minutes.
4. Combine the beans and steak sauce in a small bowl, stir to coat, and then mash with a fork.
5. Split the hamburger buns and spread the bean mixture on both sides.
6. Place the grilled mushroom on one of the prepared halves. Layer the onion, tomatoes, and lettuce on top, then press the other prepared bun half into place.

Food groups: *protein (kidney beans), carbohydrate (hamburger buns), fruit (tomato), vegetable (mushroom, onion, lettuce)*

SUGGESTED SIDE DISH: sweet potato fries (see Snacks)

HOLY LAND POTATO SALAD

Serves 6

There's a whole category of salad recipes coming up, but here's a salad I wanted to fit into the lunch category, in honor of all the afternoon church picnics I attended growing up where potato salad was ever present. Really, has there ever been a church picnic, or any other kind of picnic, without potato salad? Is that even allowed?

This righteous potato salad is dairy-free, and its Mediterranean ingredients (chickpeas, dates, balsamic vinegar, olive oil) give it special character, texture, and flavor. It is heavenly.

3 large red potatoes

1 medium red onion, chopped

1 (15-ounce) can chickpeas, rinsed and drained
¼ cup extra virgin olive oil
2 tablespoons white balsamic vinegar
Pinch of salt
1 teaspoon black pepper
5–6 dates, pitted

1. Steam or boil the potatoes until tender. Drain and let cool slightly.
2. While the potatoes are cooking, combine the onion and chickpeas in a small bowl and lightly mash with a fork or potato/bean masher.
3. In another small bowl, combine the oil, vinegar, salt, and pepper and whisk to blend.
4. When the potatoes are cooked, cut them into large chunks while still warm and combine in a large bowl with the onion-chickpea mixture. Pour the vinaigrette over the mixture. Stir well. Allow to rest until the salad cools to room temperature.
5. Roughly chop the pitted dates and stir into the salad.
6. Cover and refrigerate until ready to serve. Stir again before serving.

Food groups: protein (chickpeas), carbohydrate (potatoes), fruit (dates), vegetable (potatoes, onions)

SPRING ROLLS WITH PEANUT SAUCE

Serves 6

These are beautiful little works of culinary art, and they are easy to make. The colorful veggies shine through the translucent rice wrapping in a very eye-pleasing way. In fact, spring rolls look so wonderful that you almost don't want to eat them. But they taste wonderful, too, so go ahead!

FOR THE SPRING ROLLS:
2 ounces rice vermicelli noodles, cooked according to package instructions
½ cup baby lima beans
1 red cabbage leaf, chopped or cut into short thin slices
6 fresh basil leaves, torn in half
6 fresh mint leaves, torn in half
1 cucumber, chopped

2 scallions, chopped

1 carrot, grated

1 tablespoon fresh lime juice

6 spring roll skins (also called rice wraps; see Note)

FOR THE PEANUT SAUCE:

½ cup creamy peanut butter

¼ cup water, more if needed

1 tablespoon reduced-sodium soy sauce

1 teaspoon fresh lime juice

¼ teaspoon garlic powder

¼ teaspoon ground ginger

¼ teaspoon red pepper flakes

TO MAKE THE SPRING ROLLS:

1. In a large bowl, combine the cooked noodles, lima beans, cabbage, basil, mint, cucumber, scallions, carrot, and lime juice and mix well.
2. Dip one rice wrap in a bowl of hot water for 1 second to soften, and then lay it on a flat surface.
3. Place one-sixth of the filling across the middle of the wrap, tuck in both sides of the wrap, then roll into a log shape, enclosing the filling inside the wrap.
4. Repeat with remaining ingredients to make 6 spring rolls.

TO MAKE THE PEANUT SAUCE:

1. Combine all the ingredients in a small bowl and stir until smooth and somewhat runny. Add more water if necessary

TO SERVE:

1. Slice each spring roll into two or three pieces and serve with the peanut sauce for dipping.

Food groups: protein (lima beans, peanut sauce), carbohydrate (rice wraps, rice noodles), fruit (lime juice), vegetable (cabbage, basil, mint, cucumber, scallions, carrot)

NOTE: Spring roll skins are available in the Asian or international food aisle of most large markets.

AVOCADO TACOS WITH MEXICAN SLAW AND RED CHILE SAUCE

Serves 4

Avocado, a healthy fat from the plant world, fills in spectacularly for the animal fat found in traditional tacos. There's so much good stuff going on in these beauties, nobody's going to miss the meat and cheese. Your carnivore friends will take one bite and ask for the recipe. You watch.

FOR THE MEXICAN SLAW:

2 cups chopped cabbage (red or green or a combination of both)
½ cup chopped radish
½ cup cooked black beans
½ cup chopped onion (red or white)
¼ cup chopped carrot
¼ cup chopped fresh cilantro
1 jalapeño pepper, cored and chopped
Juice of 1 lime
2 tablespoons extra virgin olive oil
1 teaspoon white vinegar
1 tablespoon black pepper

FOR THE RED CHILE SAUCE:

1 (8-ounce) can tomato sauce
½ cup water
1 tablespoon white vinegar
1 teaspoon chile powder
1 teaspoon ground cumin
1 teaspoon onion powder
1 teaspoon garlic powder
½ teaspoon cayenne pepper
¼ teaspoon paprika

FOR ASSEMBLING THE TACOS:

8 corn tortillas
4 ripe avocados, peeled, seeded, and cut into chunks

TO MAKE THE SLAW:

1. Combine all the slaw ingredients in a large bowl and mix well. Cover and refrigerate for at least 1 hour.

TO MAKE THE CHILE SAUCE:

1. Combine all the ingredients in a saucepan over low heat and stir. Simmer, stirring frequently, for 15–20 minutes, or until thickened. Allow to cool for best flavor.

TO ASSEMBLE THE TACOS:

1. Heat the corn tortillas using one of several methods: On the stove top, heat one at a time in a dry or lightly oiled pan over medium heat for 30 seconds on each side. Or, in a 350-degree oven, place two stacks of four tortillas each, wrapped in aluminum foil, and warm for 10–15 minutes. Or, in the microwave, place two stacks of four tortillas each, wrapped in microwave-safe plastic wrap, and heat for 30 seconds, turn and heat for another 20–30 seconds. Unwrap carefully.
2. When the tortillas are prepared, load them with the avocado chunks, Mexican slaw, and red chile sauce, then fold and serve.

Food groups: protein (black beans), carbohydrate (tortillas), fruit (avocado, lime, tomato sauce), vegetable (cabbage, radish, onion, carrot, cilantro)

LOADED SWEET POTATO

Serves 1

You know the loaded potato, right? A baked spud split open and heaped with yummy stuff? Yeah, that's pretty good. But a loaded sweet potato is even better. First, a sweet potato has that hearty red color, so it's just better looking. Second, the sweet potato has a few nutritional edges over its white cousin. It has more vitamins and fiber, and fewer calories. Winner!

1 plump sweet potato, unpeeled
1 tablespoon dairy-free butter spread
½ cup cooked black beans, drained
¼ cup cooked corn kernels, drained
1 fresh scallion, chopped
¼ cup red salsa (see John's Famous All-Red Salsa, page 120)
1 tablespoon chopped fresh cilantro
¼ teaspoon red pepper flakes

1. Scrub the sweet potato, trim the ends, and remove any blemishes (you'll be eating the skin!).
2. Bake, steam, or microwave the sweet potato until cooked (see Tip).
3. Slice the cooked potato down the middle and spread open.
4. Add the dairy-free butter spread and use a fork to mash and mix it with the sweet potato flesh.
5. Spoon the beans, corn, and chopped scallion into the potato. Top with the salsa, cilantro, and red pepper flakes and serve.

Food groups: *protein (black beans), carbohydrate (sweet potato), fruit (tomato salsa), vegetable (corn, scallion, cilantro)*

....

TIP: Microwaving is the quickest way to cook a sweet potato. Just pierce the sweet potato with a sharp knife, then wrap the potato in a paper bag or damp paper towel and microwave for 5-6 minutes on full power. Allow to rest a few more minutes before unwrapping.

To bake, preheat the oven to 350 degrees, wrap the sweet potato in foil, place on a baking sheet or directly on the oven rack, and bake until tender, 50-60 minutes depending on the size of the sweet potato. Test for tenderness by piercing with a sharp knife.

To cook on the stove top, pour enough water into a cooking pot to cover the sweet potato, or, if using a steamer basket, enough water to reach the bottom of the basket. Bring the water to a boil. Add the sweet potato and boil or steam until tender, 30-40 minutes depending on the size of the sweet potato.

....

THREE AMIGOS CHILI

Serves 6-8

Who thinks vegetarian chili isn't macho? The bean brothers are in town, and they mean to prove otherwise. Pinto, kidney, and black beans band together in this fast, easy chili that will put fire to the feet of any doubters!

1 tablespoon olive oil
1 large onion, chopped
2 jalapeño peppers, cored and chopped
2 cloves garlic, minced

1 (15-ounce) can pinto beans, rinsed and drained
1 (15-ounce) can kidney beans, with juice
1 (15-ounce) can black beans, rinsed and drained
1 (16-ounce) can diced tomatoes
1 (8-ounce) can tomato sauce
1 cup tomato juice
6 tablespoons store-bought hot sauce
1 teaspoon ground cumin

1. In a large skillet, heat the olive oil over medium heat, add the chopped onion and jalapeños, and cook for 2 minutes, stirring often. Add the garlic and cook for 2 more minutes, stirring often.
2. Add the beans and stir to combine.
3. Add the diced tomatoes, tomato sauce, tomato juice, hot sauce, and cumin and stir to combine.
4. Bring to a boil, then reduce the heat to low and simmer, uncovered, for 10 minutes, stirring occasionally, until the chili is thickened. If extra thickness is desired, partially mash with a potato/bean masher.

Food groups: *protein (beans), carbohydrate (beans), fruit (tomato), vegetable (onion, jalapeño, garlic)*

DINNER

MOM'S LENTIL ROAST

Serves 12

This hearty casserole is revered in my family. It was a standard in my mom's culinary repertoire. And I know that she learned it from her mom. And today, my siblings and I carry on the tradition.

It's a tradition worth sharing. Lentil roast is great as a hot dish, scooped onto a plate and topped with mushroom gravy or salsa. We also love it cold. We'll cut rough slices to make sandwiches, layered with pickle, onion, and tomato slices on good sheepherder's bread.

4 cups cooked lentils, drained
1 large yellow or white onion, chopped
½ cup raw chopped walnuts
4 rounded tablespoons tomato paste
½ cup vegetable oil
½ cup flour
½ cup unsweetened soy milk
1 tablespoon garlic powder
¼ teaspoon ground sage
Pinch of salt
2 cups crushed corn flakes

1. Preheat the oven to 350 degrees. Coat a 2½-quart glass casserole dish (9 × 5 × 3 inches or 9 × 13 × 2 inches) with cooking spray.
2. Using a blender or food processor, combine all the ingredients and blend until smooth. If you don't have a blender, mash the lentils by hand with a potato/bean masher, mince the onion, and crush the walnuts in a paper or plastic bag using a hammer or rolling pin, then combine with the other ingredients and mix thoroughly by hand. You should end up with a batter that is dense but pliable. If it seems too dry and stiff, add a little more soy milk.
3. Spread the mixture in the prepared baking dish and bake uncovered for about 60 minutes, until firm and lightly browned around the edges.

4. Remove from the oven and allow to cool for 20–30 minutes before serving. Serve hot, topped with salsa, steak sauce, or meatless gravy. Or refrigerate and serve cold in sandwiches with pickles, onions, and tomatoes.

Food groups: protein (lentils, walnuts, soy milk), carbohydrate (corn flakes), fruit (tomato paste), vegetable (onion)

SUGGESTED SIDE DISHES: corn on the cob, mixed vegetables, fresh fruit

TIP: The classic Mom's Lentil Roast isn't glazed, but here's how to add a delicious one, if you like.

> 1 tablespoon balsamic vinegar
> 1 tablespoon maple syrup
> 3 tablespoons chili sauce (see Note)

1. Combine all the ingredients in a small bowl and whisk to blend.
2. When the lentil roast has cooked for 50 minutes, remove from the oven and top with the glaze mixture, spreading to coat evenly.
3. Return the roast to the oven and cook for 10 minutes longer, or until done.

NOTE: Chili sauce is a fancy sort of ketchup with chile peppers that is available in the condiment aisle of many large markets. If you can't find it, just use ketchup.

PIZZA ALLEGRO

Serves 4-6

I've given this recipe a jazzy Italian name, but all it really means is "fast pizza." What makes it fast? We use ready-made pizza crust, available in most large markets. Of course, if you are feeling heroic, you can make this recipe starting with good old wet pizza dough, either the kind you make from scratch or the kind you buy at the store, but that's going to take a lot longer. It will be good, for sure, but you'll have to change the name to Pizza Adagio. That's jazzy Italian for "slow pizza."

1 (12-inch) ready-made pizza crust
1 (6-ounce) can tomato paste

1 tablespoon Italian seasoning (or your own mix of ground oregano,
 rosemary, and thyme)
1 cup dairy-free parmesan substitute (store-bought or see following recipe)
½ red onion, thinly sliced
1 cup mixed fresh mushrooms, sliced or roughly chopped
1 cup chopped bell pepper (use a mix of green, red, orange, and yellow
 peppers for extra eye appeal)
½ cup sliced black olives, drained
½ cup fresh basil, roughly chopped
1 tablespoon red pepper flakes

1. Preheat the oven to 500 degrees. Coat a pizza pan or baking sheet with cooking spray.
2. Place the ready-made pizza crust on the prepared pan. In a small bowl, combine the tomato paste and Italian seasonings and spread over the pizza crust.
3. Sprinkle with one-third of the dairy-free parmesan substitute.
4. Layer the onion, mushrooms, peppers, olives, and basil on the pizza crust, and top with the remaining two-thirds of the dairy-free parmesan substitute.
5. Sprinkle with the red pepper flakes.
6. Bake for about 10 minutes, checking to avoid burning.

Food groups: *protein (dairy-free parmesan substitute), carbohydrate (pizza crust), fruit (tomato paste, olives), vegetable (onion, mushrooms, peppers, basil)*

SUGGESTED SIDE DISHES: bean salad, corn on the cob, melon slices

DAIRY-FREE PARMESAN SUBSTITUTE

Makes 1 cup

¾ cup raw cashews
3 tablespoons nutritional yeast
1 teaspoon garlic powder
½ teaspoon sea salt

Combine all the ingredients in a blender and process until a fine meal is formed.

BLACK BEAN AND BLACKENED CORN ENCHILADAS

Serves 6

Spicy black beans and flame-roasted corn kernels team up with other vegetables and herbs to make a memorable enchilada casserole. You can make the dish spicier by using more chile pepper or milder by using less.

> 3 ears fresh corn
>
> 2 (15-ounce) cans black beans, rinsed, drained, and lightly mashed with fork or potato/bean masher
>
> 1 (6-ounce) can pitted black olives, drained and roughly chopped or sliced
>
> 1 red onion, chopped
>
> 1 jalapeño pepper, cored and chopped
>
> 1 cup fresh cilantro, chopped, divided
>
> 1 tablespoon ground cumin
>
> 1 tablespoon chile powder
>
> 2 cups shredded dairy-free pepper jack cheese substitute (store-bought or see following recipe), divided
>
> 1 (28-ounce) can red enchilada sauce, divided
>
> 12 fresh corn tortillas, divided
>
> 1 tablespoon red pepper flakes

1. Preheat the oven to 350 degrees. Coat a 9 × 12-inch baking dish with cooking spray or olive oil.
2. Flame-roast the corn on the grill or stove top, turning each ear to moderately blacken the kernels on all sides. If fresh corn is unavailable, frozen or canned corn can be stir-fried in a little oil until moderately blackened.
3. Cut the blackened corn kernels from the cobs, add to a large bowl along with the beans, olives, onion, and jalapeño, and mix well.
4. Add half of the cilantro and the cumin and chile powder. Mix well again.
5. Add half of the dairy-free pepper jack shreds. Mix well again.
6. Add about 4 ounces of the enchilada sauce. Mix well until the sauce is absorbed. The resulting mixture should be thick and spoonable, not soupy.
7. Pour just enough enchilada sauce to cover the bottom of the prepared baking dish.

8. Stack 6 tortillas on a microwave-safe plate, cover with a moistened paper towel, and microwave for 30–40 seconds to soften. Repeat with the remaining 6 tortillas.

9. One at a time, spread each tortilla with a ¼ cup dollop of the bean mixture, roll up, and place carefully in the baking dish, seam side down. Arrange the enchiladas side by side as you proceed.

10. When the dish is filled, pour over the rest of the enchilada sauce and sprinkle with the rest of the dairy-free pepper jack shreds.

11. Bake uncovered for 30 minutes, or until lightly browned on top. Remove from the oven and allow to cool for 20–30 minutes.

12. Sprinkle with the red pepper flakes and the remaining cilantro.

Food groups: *protein (cheese substitute, black beans), carbohydrate (tortillas), fruit (olives), vegetable (corn, onion, jalapeño, cilantro)*

SUGGESTED SIDE DISHES: green salad, fresh fruit

DAIRY-FREE PEPPER JACK SUBSTITUTE

Makes approximately 2 cups

3 cups water, divided
1 cup raw cashews
2 teaspoons agar powder
¼ cup nutritional yeast
¼ cup fresh lemon juice
1 tablespoon onion powder
1 teaspoon garlic powder
1 teaspoon red pepper flakes
1 teaspoon black pepper
Pinch of salt

1. Bring 2 cups of the water to a boil in a small saucepan. Add the raw cashews and boil for 10 minutes to soften. Drain the cashews and set aside. Discard the water.

2. Bring the remaining 1 cup water to a boil, add the agar powder, and stir constantly until the powder dissolves completely.

3. Using a blender or food processor, combine the agar solution with the drained cashews, nutritional yeast, lemon juice, onion powder, garlic powder, red pepper flakes, black pepper, and salt and blend until thickened and smooth.
4. Pour into an oil-sprayed glass container and refrigerate until the mixture hardens into cheese form.
5. Use a spatula to carefully remove the pepper jack from the container and use a box grater to shred.

MIGHTY MUJADDARA

Serves 6–8

One of the great dishes of antiquity, mujaddara is thought to derive from the "pottage of lentils" that figures so prominently in the Bible story of Jacob and Esau. You remember the story, don't you? It seems that Esau is so famished after a hard day's work, and the stew that his younger brother Jacob is making smells so good, that Esau buys it from him, offering his birthright inheritance in exchange. Now, that's some good pottage!

The traditional recipe for mujaddara simply calls for lentils or rice, or both, and onions. I've punched it up a bit with a couple of extra ingredients.

   2 tablespoons raw pine nuts
   3 tablespoons olive oil
   5 yellow onions, chopped
   1 cup lentils, cooked
   1 cup whole-grain brown rice, cooked
   1 cup dates, seeded and chopped
   1 teaspoon salt
   ¼ cup chopped fresh cilantro

1. Toast the pine nuts by stirring constantly in a dry pan over medium heat until they just start to brown. Remove the pan immediately from the heat and continue to stir constantly for 1 minute, then pour into a shallow dish to cool.
2. In a large pan over very low heat, add the olive oil and cook the chopped onions, stirring often, until soft and sweet, about 20 minutes.
3. Add the cooked lentils, cooked rice, chopped dates, and salt and mix well.
4. Place in serving bowl and garnish with the toasted pine nuts and chopped cilantro.

Food groups: *protein (pine nuts, lentils), carbohydrate (rice), fruit (dates), vegetable (onion, cilantro)*

SUGGESTED SIDE DISHES: artichokes, roasted beets, green salad, crusty whole-grain bread

SPINACH, MUSHROOM, AND CASHEW LASAGNA

Serves 8

Mamma mia! This pasta casserole is a renaissance masterpiece. *Delizioso!*

2 cups sliced mushrooms
2 tablespoons olive oil
1 tablespoon garlic powder
1 tablespoon ground oregano
4 cups fresh baby spinach
2 fresh tomatoes
2 (24-ounce) jars meat-free, dairy-free pasta sauce, divided
9 dry lasagna noodles, divided
2 cups dairy-free ricotta cheese substitute (store-bought or see following recipe), divided
1 tablespoon red pepper flakes

1. Preheat the oven to 400 degrees. Coat a 9 × 12-inch baking dish with cooking spray.
2. Toss the mushrooms with the olive oil, garlic powder, and oregano. Add the spinach and toss again. Thickly slice the tomatoes and set aside separately.
3. Pour and spread 8 ounces of the pasta sauce to cover the bottom of the dish. Arrange 3 dry lasagna noodles in a single layer in the dish. Pour and spread 8 ounces of pasta sauce on the noodles.
4. Add half the dairy-free ricotta and half the mushroom-spinach mix. Pour and spread another 8 ounces of pasta sauce. Arrange 3 more dry lasagna noodles in a single layer. Pour and spread another 8 ounces of pasta sauce on these noodles.
5. Add the remaining dairy-free ricotta and the remaining mushroom-spinach mix. Pour and spread another 8 ounces of pasta sauce. Arrange the remaining 3 dry lasagna noodles in a single layer on top. Pour and spread the remaining 8 ounces pasta sauce to cover. Top with a single layer of fresh tomato slices.

6. Cover with foil and bake for 40 minutes. Remove the foil and bake for 20 minutes longer.

7. Remove from the oven, sprinkle with the red pepper flakes, and allow to cool for 20–30 minutes before serving.

Food groups: protein (spinach, dairy-free ricotta cheese substitute), carbohydrate (pasta), fruit (tomatoes), vegetable (mushrooms, spinach)

SUGGESTED SIDE DISHES: artichokes, green salad, fresh fruit

DAIRY-FREE RICOTTA CHEESE SUBSTITUTE

Makes 2 cups

2 cups water
2 cups raw cashews
Pinch of salt
1 teaspoon black pepper
3 tablespoons nutritional yeast
1 tablespoon cider vinegar

1. Bring the water to a boil in a small saucepan, add the raw cashews, and simmer for 10 minutes to soften.

2. Drain the cashews, reserving the water.

3. Season the drained cashews with the salt, pepper, and nutritional yeast.

4. Using a blender or food processor, combine the seasoned cashews with the cider vinegar, and ½ cup of the reserved cashew water, and blend until thick and creamy. Add more of the reserved cashew water to get the desired consistency.

ELLEN G. WHITE'S FAVORITE NOODLE DISH: BAKED MACARONI AND CORN CASSEROLE

Serves 6

We have my Auntie Grace to thank for much of the family's oldest culinary lore, stretching all the way back to the time of Ellen G. White. Grace White Jacques was my grandfather's sister, which means she was my grand-aunt, but we all called her Auntie Grace.

She had grown up in the actual company of Ellen G. White, her grandmother, and had spent countless hours in the Elmshaven kitchen and dining room. She told many stories about her grandmother's favorite foods, recipes, and eating habits.

Ellen G. White ate only two main meals a day—breakfast and an afternoon meal that was called dinner. One of her "dinner" favorites was a baked macaroni and corn dish that was vegetarian, but definitely not vegan. It was loaded with dairy milk, butter, and cheese. Turning it vegan is an easy trick, though. You'll see.

½ cup dairy-free butter spread
1 cup unsweetened almond milk
½ cup nutritional yeast
1 teaspoon garlic powder
1 teaspoon ground turmeric
Pinch of salt
6 cups cooked macaroni noodles
1 (15-ounce) can whole-kernel corn, mostly drained but reserving a little of
    the juice
1 (15-ounce) can creamed corn
½ cup fresh basil leaves, sliced or chopped

1. Preheat the oven to 350 degrees. Coat a 9 × 13 baking dish with cooking spray.
2. In a saucepan, melt the dairy-free butter spread over low heat. Add the almond milk and whisk for about 2 minutes until the mixture reaches a light simmer.
3. Add the nutritional yeast, garlic powder, turmeric, and salt and whisk until thickened. Don't allow to boil (reduce the heat, if necessary). When the sauce has thickened, remove from the heat.
4. In a mixing bowl, combine the cooked noodles, the whole-kernel corn with a little of its juice, the creamed corn, and the sauce. Mix well.
5. Pour the noodle and corn mixture into the prepared baking dish and bake uncovered for 30–40 minutes until lightly browned.
6. Remove from the oven, sprinkle with the fresh basil, and serve hot.

Food groups: protein (almond milk, nutritional yeast), carbohydrate (pasta), vegetable (corn, basil)

SUGGESTED SIDE DISHES: green salad, fresh fruit

LAYERED EGGPLANT, ZUCCHINI, AND TOMATO CASSEROLE

Serves 6

This hearty casserole is stuffed with garden goodness. Serve it with garlicky smashed potatoes for a meal to remember.

3 or 4 medium zucchini, sliced lengthwise ¼ inch thick

2 or 3 long, narrow eggplants, peeled and sliced lengthwise ⅓ inch thick

4 tablespoons olive oil, divided

Salt and black pepper

1 medium onion, finely chopped

1 pound plum tomatoes, chopped

¾ cup crumbled dairy-free feta cheese substitute (store-bought or see following recipe), divided

½ cup chopped fresh basil, divided

½ cup dry bread crumbs

1. Preheat the oven to 425 degrees. Coat 2 rimmed baking sheets and a 9 × 13-inch baking dish with cooking spray.
2. Brush the zucchini and eggplant slices with 1 tablespoon of the olive oil, and season with salt and pepper.
3. Place the zucchini slices on one baking sheet and the eggplant slices on the other baking sheet, arranging the slices so they slightly overlap each other. Bake for 15 minutes, or until tender.
4. In a large skillet, heat 2 tablespoons of the olive oil, add the chopped onion, and cook until softened, about 3 minutes.
5. Add the tomatoes and cook for 1–2 minutes, until bubbling. Season with salt and pepper.
6. Arrange half the eggplant slices side by side in the prepared baking dish and spread a quarter of the tomato-onion mixture on top.
7. Create a new layer by arranging half the zucchini slices side by side and topping with another quarter of the tomato-onion mixture.
8. Sprinkle half of the dairy-free feta cheese substitute and half of the basil on top.
9. Layer the remaining eggplant slices and top with another quarter of the tomato-onion mixture.

10. Layer the remaining zucchini slices and top with the remaining quarter of the tomato-onion mixture.
11. Top with the remaining dairy-free feta cheese substitute and the remaining basil.
12. Mix the bread crumbs with the remaining 1 tablespoon olive oil and sprinkle over the top.
13. Bake uncovered for 25–30 minutes until bubbling and crisp. Remove from the oven and allow to cool 20 minutes before serving.

Food groups: protein (dairy-free feta cheese substitute), carbohydrate (bread crumbs), fruit (tomato), vegetable (zucchini, eggplant, onion, basil)

SUGGESTED SIDE DISHES: wild rice or garlicky smashed potatoes (stir crushed roasted garlic into mashed potatoes and top with pine nuts and chopped chives)

DAIRY-FREE FETA CHEESE SUBSTITUTE

Makes 1–1½ cups

1½ cups almond meal
¼ cup water
¼ cup lemon juice
3 tablespoons olive oil
1 tablespoon garlic powder

1. Preheat the oven to 350 degrees. Coat a baking sheet with cooking spray or line with parchment paper.
2. Using a food processor or blender, combine all the ingredients and blend for 3–5 minutes to form a smooth paste.
3. Turn out the mixture onto a sheet of plastic wrap. Gather up the plastic wrap around the mixture and twist the top of the wrap to shape the mixture into a firm round loaf about 1¼ inches thick.
4. Unwrap the loaf and place on the prepared baking sheet.
5. Bake for about 20 minutes, until the surface is crusty and slightly golden.
6. Remove from the oven and allow to cool completely. Use a fork to loosely crumble before use.

SALADS

SNAP PEA SALAD WITH PECANS AND CRANBERRIES

Serves 6

You'll have this recipe memorized before too long. You're going to make it that often. It's so pretty, so delicious, so refreshing. Your loved ones and friends will be asking for the recipe. Constantly. Good thing you'll have it memorized!

⅔ cup raw pecan halves
1 cup extra virgin olive oil, divided
1 tablespoon sugar
Pinch of salt
1 pound snap peas
¼ cup balsamic vinegar
½ cup dried cranberries

1. Preheat the oven to 325 degrees.
2. In a small bowl, combine the pecans with ¼ cup of the olive oil, sugar, and salt, and stir to coat. Spread on a baking sheet and bake for 15 minutes. Remove from the heat and stir.
3. Trim the stem and remove the string from each snap pea, then slice each snap pea on the diagonal into several pieces.
4. Bring a saucepan of water to a boil, add the snap peas to the water, and cook for 1 minute.
5. Drain the snap peas, rinse in cold water, and then pat dry with a towel.
6. In a small bowl, whisk the remaining ¾ cup olive oil and the vinegar to make a vinaigrette.
7. Combine the pecans, snap peas, cranberries, and vinaigrette in salad bowl and mix well.

Food groups: *protein (pecans), carbohydrate (sugar), fruit (dried cranberries), vegetable (snap peas)*

EMPIRE SALAD

Serves 6

I invented this recipe to honor Southern California's agriculturally bountiful Inland Empire, east of Los Angeles, where I have lived for most of my life. The recipe appears in the 2010 book *City of San Bernardino Bicentennial Cookbook*.

Empire Salad is an attractive mix of ingredients that have historical importance in the region. There are oranges, in celebration of San Bernardino's century-old National Orange Show and the endless miles of orange groves that once dominated the local landscape. There are grapes, a nod to the Cucamonga Valley, which is California's oldest wine country. There is lemon, in tribute to Upland's annual Lemon Festival, and cherries, a salute to Cherry Valley's annual Cherry Festival. There are green olives, a compliment to the famous Graber Olives that trace their origin to Ontario, California. And there are almonds, to commemorate the fact that pioneer growers in the San Gorgonio Pass helped form the 1910 cooperative that became Blue Diamond Growers, the world's largest tree nut production and marketing company.

⅓ cup sliced raw almonds
1 (12-ounce) bag romaine lettuce hearts, chopped
1 (12-ounce) bag baby spinach leaves
½ red onion, thinly sliced
24 green olives, pitted and cut in half
24 fresh seedless grapes, cut in half
3 tablespoons extra virgin olive oil
1 tablespoon salad vinegar
3 tablespoons fresh lemon juice
1 tablespoon sugar
Pinch of salt
1 teaspoon black pepper
4 navel oranges, peeled, sectioned, and cut into ½-inch pieces, with juice reserved
1 pound frozen pitted cherries, thawed but still cold

1. Toast the sliced almonds by stirring constantly in a dry pan over medium heat until they just start to brown. Remove the pan immediately from the heat and continue to stir constantly for 1 minute, then pour into a shallow dish to cool.

2. In a large bowl, combine the lettuce, spinach, onion, olives, and grapes.
3. In a small bowl, whisk the olive oil, vinegar, lemon juice, reserved orange juice, sugar, salt, and pepper. Add the dressing to the bowl, tossing to coat.
4. Drain cherries, if necessary, and scatter on top.
5. Scatter the orange pieces on top of the cherries.
6. Scatter most or all of the toasted almonds on top of the salad, without overly obscuring the fruit, and serve.

Food groups: *protein (almonds), carbohydrate (sugar), fruit (oranges, cherries, olives, grapes, lemon juice), vegetable (lettuce, spinach, onion)*

ELLEN G. WHITE'S FAVORITE SALAD: CUCUMBER, RADISH, AND TURNIP SALAD

Serves 4–6

My great-great-grandmother loved greens, vegetables, and fruits, so it's no surprise that she was a big fan of salads. Interestingly, she didn't like to mix vegetables and fruits at the same meal, so typically she would have her fruit salad in the mornings or as an evening treat, and her vegetable salad in the afternoon. A special favorite was a salad of cucumbers, radishes, and turnips. We are indebted to my Auntie Grace for this little family secret. She once drew up a list of Ellen G. White's favorite foods, and this salad is one of the standouts.

> 3 fresh cucumbers, unpeeled and sliced
> 6 fresh red radishes, unpeeled and sliced
> 2 turnips, unpeeled and grated
> 1 cup chopped green cabbage
> ⅓ cup fresh dill, minced
> Pinch of salt
> 6 tablespoons extra virgin olive oil
> 2 tablespoons white wine vinegar
> ⅓ cup sliced almonds, raw or toasted

1. In a serving bowl, combine the cucumbers, radishes, turnips, cabbage, and dill with a pinch of salt and stir to mix.
2. In a small bowl, whisk the oil and vinegar, drizzle over the salad, and stir lightly to mix.

3. Garnish with the sliced almonds. To toast almonds, stir constantly in a dry pan over medium heat until they just start to brown.

Food groups: protein (almonds), vegetable (cucumbers, radishes, turnips, cabbage, dill)

TRIPLE SLAW

Serves 6–8

This recipe combines three cabbage varieties plus other goodies to create a refreshing coleslaw that is off the charts in good looks and good flavors.

½ head green cabbage, shredded
½ head Napa or Chinese cabbage, shredded
½ head red cabbage, shredded
½ yellow or orange bell pepper, cored, seeded, and sliced into thin strips
½ red bell pepper, cored, seeded, and sliced into thin strips
½ cup chopped scallions
½ cup chopped fresh cilantro
½ cup chopped pineapple
¼ cup sliced almonds, raw or toasted
¼ cup extra virgin olive oil
2 tablespoons white wine vinegar
1 tablespoon sugar
Pinch of salt
1 teaspoon black pepper

1. In a large bowl, combine the cabbages, bell peppers, scallions, cilantro, pineapple, and sliced almonds. To toast almonds, stir constantly in a dry pan over medium heat until they just start to brown.
2. In a small bowl, whisk the olive oil, vinegar, sugar, and salt, add to the slaw, and toss well to mix.
3. Sprinkle the black pepper over the top.

Food groups: protein (almonds), carbohydrate (sugar), fruit (pineapple), vegetable (cabbage, bell pepper, scallions, cilantro)

CREAMY BROCCOLI SALAD

Serves 8

This salad has made appearances at many a picnic or party where I have been a witness to its crowd-gathering power. The bowl always ends up empty, and everyone wants the recipe. Here it is.

  2 large heads fresh raw broccoli, cut into florets
  1 cup dried cranberries
  ½ small red onion, chopped
  ½ cup chopped celery
  1 cup shelled pecans, broken into pieces of various size, divided
  1 cup dairy-free mayonnaise
  ¼ cup sugar
  ¼ cup apple cider vinegar

1. Combine the broccoli, cranberries, onion, celery, and half the pecan pieces in a large bowl and mix well.
2. In a small bowl, whisk the dairy-free mayonnaise, sugar, and vinegar and pour over the broccoli mixture. Mix well again.
3. Sprinkle with the remaining pecan pieces.

Food groups: protein (pecans), carbohydrate (sugar), fruit (cranberries), vegetable (broccoli, onion, celery)

FARRO AND BEET SALAD

Serves 6

Farro is an ancient and venerated grain that is full of nutty, chewy goodness. In this recipe, it pairs wonderfully with the earthy taste of beets to make a memorable salad. Farro can be found in many large markets, most health food stores, and online.

  3 medium-size fresh whole beets
  3 cups water
  1 cup farro
  3 tablespoons extra virgin olive oil

Pinch of salt

1 tablespoon lemon juice

3 cloves garlic, minced

1 cup chopped fresh radicchio

1 cup seeded and chopped fresh cucumber

½ cup chopped red onion

½ cup chopped fresh parsley

¼ cup sunflower seeds, raw or roasted

1. Trim the ends of the beets and steam or boil for about 35 minutes, or until tender (a sharp knife should pass easily through the heart of the beet). Remove from the heat, drain if necessary, and set aside to cool.
2. Bring the water to a boil in a saucepan, rinse the farro, add to the boiling water, reduce the heat to low, and simmer for 30 minutes, until tender. Drain any remaining water.
3. Add the olive oil, salt, lemon juice, and garlic to the hot farro and stir well to mix. Set aside to cool.
4. Peel the cooled beets and cut into wedges.
5. Combine the radicchio, cucumber, onion, and cooked farro in a serving dish and stir to mix.
6. Top with the beet wedges and sprinkle with the parsley and sunflower seeds.

Food groups: protein (sunflower seeds), carbohydrate (farro), fruit (lemon juice), vegetable (beets, radicchio, cucumber, onion, parsley)

MEDITERRANEAN WHEAT SALAD

Serves 6

This chilled wheat salad is bejeweled with colorful confetti-cut veggies and golden toasted sesame seeds. Chickpeas and herbs add savory goodness, and a splash each of olive oil and lemon juice makes it zing.

Once it's on the table, take a moment to admire it before everyone plunges in.

2 cups uncooked whole-grain bulgur wheat

2 tablespoons toasted sesame seeds

½ red onion, diced

1 red bell pepper, cored, seeded, and diced
1 unpeeled cucumber, seeded and diced
1 unpeeled yellow squash, seeded and diced
1 carrot, peeled and grated
1 (15-ounce) can chickpeas, rinsed and drained
½ cup fresh dill, minced
½ cup fresh parsley, minced
4 cloves garlic, minced
½ cup fresh lemon juice
½ cup extra virgin olive oil
Pinch of salt
½ cup fresh pomegranate arils (seeds), for garnish (optional)

1. Cook the bulgur wheat according to package directions, or add the bulgur wheat to 4 cups water in a large pan. Bring to a boil, reduce the heat to low, tilt the lid, and simmer for 15–20 minutes. Drain any remaining water, allow the wheat to cool slightly, and then fluff with a fork.

2. Toast sesame seeds. Stir constantly in a dry pan over medium heat until they just start to brown. In a mixing bowl, combine the wheat with all the remaining ingredients, except for the optional pomegranate arils, and stir well. Refrigerate until chilled.

3. Stir again, transfer to serving bowl, sprinkle with the pomegranate arils, if desired, and serve cold.

Food groups: *protein (chickpeas, sesame seeds), carbohydrate (bulgur wheat), fruit (lemon juice, pomegranate), vegetable (onion, bell pepper, cucumber, squash, carrot, dill, parsley, garlic.)*

....

NOTE: For a gluten-free version, use whole-grain quinoa, brown rice, or buckwheat instead of wheat.

....

SNACKS

BLACK OLIVE CAVIAR

Makes about 1½ cups

Here's a classy treat that looks like a million bucks. Actually, though, it's cheap and easy. Let's keep this a secret among ourselves, all right?

1 cup pitted chopped black olives
5 tablespoons crushed walnuts
¼ cup dried black currants
3 tablespoons fresh thyme leaves, minced
2 teaspoons chia seeds
3 tablespoons olive oil

Add all the ingredients to a bowl and mix well.

Food groups: *protein (walnuts), carbohydrate (chia seeds), fruit (olives, currants), vegetable (thyme)*

TIP: Serve on whole-grain crackers, crostini, or roasted potato slices. Can also be used as a topping on whole baked potatoes.

TOMATO TOAST TAPAS

Serves 6–8

This recipe has very few ingredients, so each one is important. Above all, the tomatoes must be ripe and full of flavor. Honestly, if you can't find fresh tomatoes that taste good, I'd rather have you make these tapas with canned tomato paste, which at least comes from tomatoes that were processed and canned at their peak. Don't worry, your tapas will be good. But trust me, if you use fresh garden-ripe tomatoes that taste sublime, your tapas will be out of this world.

2 large, flavorful beefsteak tomatoes
½ cup extra virgin olive oil, divided
Pinch of salt

1 large loaf rustic-style bread (such as ciabatta)
3 cloves fresh garlic, cut in half
⅓ cup raw pine nuts
⅓ cup fresh basil or thyme, minced

1. Preheat the oven to 350 degrees.
2. Using a sharp knife, slit the skin of each tomato in two or three places. Immerse the tomatoes in enough boiling water to cover. When the tomatoes begin to blister and shed their skin (30–40 seconds), remove with a slotted spoon and plunge into cold water. Pull away the loose skin from each tomato. Finely chop the peeled tomatoes, draining excess juice. Place in a bowl.
3. Add ¼ cup of the olive oil and a little salt to the tomatoes and stir to mix. Set aside.
4. Slice the bread loaf in half horizontally, and then cut each half crosswise into slices 1–2 inches thick.
5. Arrange the bread slices in a single layer on a baking sheet. Drizzle with the remaining ¼ cup olive oil.
6. Bake for 10–15 minutes, or until crisp and golden brown.
7. Remove from the oven and rub the bread slices with the cut garlic.
8. Spread each slice with the tomato mixture and sprinkle with the pine nuts.
9. Garnish with minced basil or thyme.

Food groups: *protein (pine nuts), carbohydrate (bread), fruit (tomato), vegetable (basil or thyme, garlic)*

NUTTY HUMMUS

Serves 4

I love traditional hummus, the Mediterranean dip made with chickpeas, lemon juice, garlic, olive oil, and tahini. Tahini, if you're not familiar with it, is like peanut butter only it's made from sesame seeds. It's very delicious and I'm always running out of it. That's why I had to create Nutty Hummus one day when I was caught short of tahini. As it turns out, peanut butter does a fine job, and it comes with plenty of its own oil, so it takes the place of both the tahini and the olive oil in the traditional hummus recipe.

1 (15-ounce) can chickpeas, mostly drained but reserving a little of the juice
Juice of 1 small lemon

1 tablespoon garlic powder
4 rounded tablespoons peanut butter
2 tablespoons chopped sun-dried tomato
1 teaspoon red pepper flakes
Crackers and veggie sticks, for serving

1. In a bowl, roughly mash the chickpeas with fork. Add the lemon juice and mix well. Add the garlic powder and mix well.
2. Add peanut butter and mix well. (If the peanut butter is refrigerated and stiff, soften it first by heating in the microwave for 20 seconds.) Add chopped sun-dried tomatoes and mix well.
3. Place the well-mixed hummus in a serving bowl and sprinkle with the red pepper flakes.
4. Serve with sturdy whole-grain crackers and fresh veggie sticks, such as carrot, celery, cucumber, zucchini, jicama, and bell pepper. Raw broccoli and cauliflower florets also work well.

Food groups: protein (chickpeas, peanut butter), carbohydrate (crackers), fruit (lemon juice, tomato), vegetable (veggie sticks)

PRAJNA POPCORN

Serves 8

Prajna is a word used in yoga and meditation to describe the inward spiritual journey toward enlightenment. Now, seriously, can popcorn help on a quest for enlightenment? Well, try this recipe and find out! Even if it isn't a round-trip ticket to nirvana and back, it's a tasty snack that will make you feel as happy as a Buddha.

½ cup unsweetened coconut flakes
1 cup salted peanut halves
1 cup wasabi peas (dried green peas coated with wasabi)
2 tablespoons curry powder
1 tablespoon ginger powder
¼ cup organic virgin coconut oil
1 tablespoon fresh lime juice
8 cups popped popcorn, prepared in a hot-air popper or pan-cooked using oil, not butter

1. Toast the coconut flakes by stirring constantly in a dry pan over medium heat until they just start to brown. Remove the pan immediately from the heat, and continue to stir constantly for 1 minute, then pour into a shallow dish to cool.
2. Combine the peanuts, wasabi peas, curry powder, and ginger powder in a large bowl and stir to mix. Add the toasted coconut flakes and stir again.
3. Warm the coconut oil in the microwave oven or on the stove top in a small pan and stir in the lime juice to mix.
4. Add the freshly popped popcorn to a large mixing bowl. Add the coconut oil and lime juice mixture and stir or shake well to mix.
5. Add the seasoned peanut, pea, and coconut flake mixture and stir or shake well to mix.

Food groups: protein (peanuts), carbohydrate (popcorn), fruit (lime juice, coconut), vegetable (peas)

STICKS

Makes about 36 sticks

These wheat snacks aren't really cookies, and they aren't really crackers. We called them Sticks in my family. Mom made them all the time. I used to think she invented them, but then I found out that her own mother made them back in the day, and I'll bet her mother's mother made them, too. There's nothing fancy about them—just a basic dough cut into stick shapes and then baked. But they are dense, chewy, satisfying, and filling, which means they really do the trick when you need a healthy, fortifying snack. They're great for lunchboxes, backpacks, and travel totes. Mom always made them with wheat flour, but I've also made them with gluten-free oat flour and quinoa flour, and they turn out very well. Good news for anyone with gluten allergy issues.

    4 cups whole-grain wheat flour
    ½ tablespoon baking powder
    2 tablespoons brown sugar
    1 teaspoon salt
    2 cups soy milk
    ½ cup vegetable oil

1. Preheat the oven to 350 degrees.
2. Combine the flour, baking powder, brown sugar, and salt in a bowl.
3. In another bowl, whisk the soy milk and oil, add to the dry ingredients, and stir to combine.

4. Coat your hands with flour to avoid sticking. Using your hands, work the mixture to form a dough, and knead it for 3 minutes or until stiff. Add a little more soy milk if too dry, or flour if too wet.

5. Place the dough on a floured surface and roll it out to a thickness of ½ inch or less. Use a knife or pizza cutter to cut into sticks that are about ½ inch wide and about 4 inches long.

6. Place sticks on a baking sheet ¼ inch apart. Bake for 30–40 minutes, or until they are firm and beginning to brown.

Food groups: *protein (soy milk), carbohydrate (flour, brown sugar)*

HUFFIN' AND PUFFIN' MUFFINS

Makes 24 mini-muffins

Yes, you'll be huffin' and puffin' after you eat one of these fiery mini-muffins. And then you'll reach for another one, because they taste so good. Of course, you can control the heat level by making them with more or less of the pepper sauce, but go on, be brave. They're good for you. This recipe calls for only two ingredients, both available at many large markets, most health food stores, and online.

1 (16-ounce) package dairy-free cornbread mix
1 (7-ounce) can chipotle peppers in adobo sauce

1. Preheat the oven according to the cornbread package directions. Coat a mini-muffin tin with cooking spray.

2. Prepare the cornbread batter following package directions. Pour the adobo sauce from the chipotle peppers into the batter and mix well. The peppers can be saved for another use or discarded.

3. Divide the cornbread batter among the prepared mini-muffin cups. Follow the package directions to bake the mini-muffins until done. Remove from the oven and allow to cool slightly before removing from the tin.

Food groups: *protein (peanut butter, if used), carbohydrate (cornbread), fruit (salsa, if used), vegetable (chile pepper sauce)*

TIP: Spread the muffins with peanut butter or dairy-free butter spread. Or drizzle with maple syrup. Or enjoy with salsa.

SWEET POTATO FRIES

Serves 4

These blushing beauties have a fancier look than plain old french fries. They have a yummier taste, too, with a sweetness that simple spuds can't deliver. Just try this recipe, and you'll have a whole new answer for that old question: "Want fries with that?"

4 sweet potatoes
3 tablespoons extra virgin olive oil
1 tablespoon garlic powder
1 teaspoon paprika

1. Preheat the oven to 400 degrees. Coat a baking sheet with cooking spray.
2. Peel and cut the sweet potatoes into french fry–style sticks.
3. Combine the oil, garlic powder, and paprika in a large bowl. Add the sweet potato fries and toss to coat in the oil-and-spice mixture.
4. Spread the sweet potato fries on the prepared baking sheet and bake for about 20 minutes, turning once, until golden brown.

Food group: *carbohydrate (sweet potato)*

DESSERTS

DARK CHOCOLATE FONDUE

Serves 8–10

Sounds decadent, doesn't it? But wait, dark chocolate is actually good for us. It's an anti-inflammatory that promotes cardiovascular health and helps keep the immune system strong. So, come on, eat dark chocolate. It's your duty!

Here's a fantastic way to perform your duty properly. Get a nice hot pot of melted dark chocolate going, and then use it for dipping nutritious fruits and even vegetables. Wait, is this even dessert anymore? It's more like health food!

Almost any fruit will work, either in chunk form or threaded onto kebab sticks. Banana chunks, strawberries, pineapple, orange segments, apple slices, long-stemmed cherries, kiwi chunks, melon and mango, peach and pear ... the list goes on. Good veggie choices include sweet bell pepper slices, whole radishes, snow peas, cucumber slices, chunks of jicama ... again, the list is long. Get going!

1 cup shredded coconut (sweetened or unsweetened)
¾ cup soy milk
1 teaspoon vanilla extract
12 ounces dairy-free dark chocolate chips (or baking bar broken into chips)

1. Toast the coconut either in a dry pan over medium heat, stirring often until the coconut is mostly golden brown, or on a baking sheet in a 350-degree oven for about 10 minutes, until the coconut is mostly golden brown. In either case, remove from the heat immediately and transfer to a shallow dish to cool. Sweetened coconut will toast more quickly than unsweetened coconut.

2. In a small pan, combine the soy milk, vanilla, and dark chocolate and stir over low heat until the chocolate just starts to melt. Remove from the heat and continue to stir until the chocolate is completely melted and the mixture is well blended and smooth.

3. Pour the chocolate mixture into a flame-heated fondue pot or a microwave-safe serving bowl that can be reheated in the microwave as necessary. Serve the toasted coconut flakes in individual finger bowls for use as a topping.

Food groups: *protein (soy milk), carbohydrate (dark chocolate), fruit (fruits for dipping, coconut), vegetable (veggies for dipping)*

TIP: Serve with fruit, veggies, and/or graham crackers for dipping.

PEACH AND RHUBARB COBBLER

Serves 6

Don't let peach season slip by without making this delicious dessert a time or two (or three or four!). And here's good news for the rest of the year: When fresh peaches are hard to find, you can prepare this dish with frozen peaches and rhubarb. Just rinse briefly under cold water to soften.

2 cups cut-up fresh peaches
2 cups cut-up fresh rhubarb
½ cup packed light brown sugar, divided
1 cup raw old-fashioned (rolled) oats
½ cup raw pecan pieces
¼ cup vegetable oil

1. Preheat the oven to 350 degrees. Coat an 8 × 8-inch baking dish with cooking spray.
2. Place the peaches and rhubarb in the prepared baking dish and toss with ¼ cup of the light brown sugar.
3. In a mixing bowl, combine the oats, pecans, vegetable oil, and remaining ¼ cup brown sugar and mix well. Spread in an even layer on top of the peach and rhubarb mixture.
4. Bake for about 45 minutes, or until the fruit is bubbling and the topping is golden brown.
5. Remove from the oven and allow to cool for 20 minutes before serving.

Food groups: *protein (pecans), carbohydrate (oats), fruit (peaches), vegetable (rhubarb)*

BEAUTIFUL BLUEBERRY SORBET

Serves 6

This is a perfect summer treat—icy cold, refreshing, and delicious. Actually, it tastes so good, you could whip up a batch in the dead of winter and nobody would blame you.

4 cups fresh or frozen blueberries

1 (6-ounce) can frozen apple juice concentrate

⅓ cup crushed pistachios

¼ cup fresh mint, minced

1. Using a blender or food processor, blend the blueberries and apple juice concentrate until liquefied.
2. Pour into 7 × 11-inch baking pan or glass casserole dish.
3. Cover and freeze until firm around the edges, about 2 hours.
4. Break the frozen mixture into pieces. Using a blender or food processor, blend the frozen pieces until smooth but not liquefied.
5. Spoon into a 5 × 9-inch loaf pan. Cover and freeze until firm.
6. Spoon into serving dishes and garnish with the crushed pistachios and fresh mint.

Food groups: protein (pistachios), carbohydrate (apple juice), fruit (blueberry, apple juice), vegetable (mint)

ELLEN G. WHITE'S FAVORITE DESSERT: BREAD PUDDING WITH RAISINS

Serves 6–8

As I said before, my great-great-grandmother didn't follow a traditional regimen of breakfast, lunch, and dinner. She ate breakfast, then an afternoon meal that she called dinner, and then nothing in the evening except a light snack—usually fruit, or nuts, or a small dessert. According to my Auntie Grace, she was very fond of bread pudding with raisins. It's an old-fashioned classic and the traditional recipe calls for lots of dairy, including milk and butter, and eggs, but it's quite easy to make a dairy-free version that tastes every bit as good.

2 cups soy milk

¼ cup dairy-free butter spread

½ cup applesauce

½ cup sugar

1 teaspoon ground cinnamon

Pinch of salt

1 teaspoon baking powder

6 slices soft bread, cut into cubes

½ cup raisins

1. Preheat the oven to 350 degrees.
2. In a 2-quart saucepan, heat the soy milk and dairy-free butter spread over medium heat until the butter spread is melted.
3. In a large bowl, combine the applesauce, sugar, cinnamon, salt, and baking powder. Add the bread cubes and raisins, and stir to mix. Add the soy milk mixture and stir to combine.
4. Pour into an ungreased 9-inch round baking pan.
5. Bake uncovered for 40–45 minutes, or until a knife inserted 1 inch from the edge comes out clean. Serve warm.

Food groups: *protein (soy milk), carbohydrate (bread), fruit (applesauce, raisins)*

CHERRY CHA-CHA

Serves 6

An upside-down graham cracker crust adds crunch to this yummy variation on cherry pie. Graham crackers go way back in the Seventh-day Adventist history books. Though the simple, wholesome crackers were invented by a Presbyterian minister, Sylvester Graham, in the 1830s, they were popularized a few decades later by the Adventist doctor John Harvey Kellogg, pioneering director of the church's world-famous Battle Creek Sanitarium in Michigan. Graham crackers were a staple on the Battle Creek menu, along with a product invented by Kellogg and his brother Will—Kellogg's Corn Flakes.

FOR THE GRAHAM CRACKER CRUST:

¼ cup dairy-free butter spread
1 cup crushed graham crackers
3 tablespoons confectioners' sugar

FOR THE CHERRY FILLING:

½ cup granulated sugar
2 tablespoons cornstarch
¼ cup cold water
¼ cup orange juice
1 pound frozen pitted Bing cherries, thawed
½ teaspoon orange zest

TO MAKE THE CRUST:

1. Melt the dairy-free butter spread in a microwave-safe bowl. Add the crushed graham crackers and confectioners' sugar and stir to combine.
2. Press the mixture into the bottom of an 8-inch square baking dish.
3. Heat for 2 minutes in the microwave or 8 minutes in a 350-degree oven. Allow to cool.

TO MAKE THE CHERRY FILLING:

1. In a saucepan, whisk together the granulated sugar and cornstarch.
2. Stir in the cold water and orange juice and bring to a boil over medium-high heat, whisking until thickened.
3. Stir in the cherries and orange zest, return to a boil, reduce the heat to low, and simmer for 10 minutes. Allow to cool.

TO ASSEMBLE:

1. Pour the cherries over the graham cracker crust and spread to cover. Place in the refrigerator and allow to chill for 3–4 hours or overnight.

Food groups: *carbohydrate (crackers), fruit (cherries, orange)*

SAVORY BAKED APPLES

Serves 4

This is an awesome dish in autumn when apples are fresh off the tree. On the other hand, it's pretty awesome any time of the year. Best apples for baking: Granny Smith, Fuji, and Rome Beauty.

¼ cup chopped raw pecans
4 large apples
½ yellow onion, finely chopped
¼ cup dairy-free butter spread
½ cup sugar
1 teaspoon ground cinnamon

1. Preheat the oven to 375 degrees.

2. Toast the chopped pecans by stirring constantly in a dry pan over medium heat until they just start to brown. Remove the pan immediately from the heat, and continue to stir constantly for 1 minute. Then pour into a shallow dish to cool.

3. Core the apples from top to near bottom, leaving enough flesh at the bottom to contain the filling.

4. Combine the pecans, dairy-free butter spread, sugar, and cinnamon in a small bowl and mix. Use this mixture to tightly fill the cavity of each apple.

5. Place apples upright in a baking dish that contains a little water, enough to cover the bottom.

6. Bake for 1 hour, or until the apples are soft and the filling is browned.

Food groups: protein (pecans), carbohydrate (sugar), fruit (apples), vegetable (onion)

STICKY RICE WITH MANGO

Serves 6

When I started loving Thai cuisine, many years ago, this was one of the reasons. What a dessert! Pairing voluptuous mango fruit with sweetened rice is pure genius. Many of the recipes for sticky rice with mango are quite complicated, but this one is easy, and the results are spectacular.

1 cup uncooked white jasmine rice
2 (13-ounce) cans coconut milk, divided
1 cup sugar, divided
2 tablespoons toasted sesame seeds
2 fresh mangoes, peeled, pitted, and chunked or sliced

1. Cook the rice according to package directions but using 1 can of the coconut milk instead of water and adding ½ cup of the sugar. The rice should be cooked until the liquid is absorbed.

2. In a separate pan, combine the remaining 1 can coconut milk and remaining ½ cup sugar, bring to a boil, and cook for about 2 minutes, stirring often, until it forms a thick, syrupy sauce.

3. Divide the rice among individual serving bowls, drizzle with the sauce, sprinkle with the toasted sesame seeds, and then arrange the mango pieces on top or to the side of each dish.

Food groups: carbohydrate (rice, sugar), fruit (coconut milk, mango)

Recommended Reading/Viewing

I have gained much insight and inspiration from the following books and video documentaries, and I recommend them wholeheartedly:

Books

The Blue Zones by Dan Buettner (National Geographic, 2008)

Breaking the Food Seduction by Neal Barnard (St. Martin's Griffin, 2004)

The China Study by T. Colin Campbell and Thomas M. Campbell II (BenBella Books, 2006)

Dreamland: Adventures in the Strange Science of Sleep by David K. Randall (W.W. Norton & Company, 2013)

Eat More, Weigh Less by Dean Ornish (HarperTorch, 2002)

Eat to Live by Joel Fuhrman (Little, Brown and Company, 2011)

The End of Diabetes by Joel Fuhrman (HarperOne, 2014)

The Engine 2 Diet by Rip Esselstyn (Grand Central Life & Style, 2009)

The Food Revolution by John Robbins (Conari Press, 2010)

The Healthiest Diet on the Planet by John McDougall and Mary McDougall (HarperOne, 2016)

Prevent and Reverse Heart Disease by Caldwell B. Esselstyn Jr. (Avery, 2007)

The Secret Life of Sleep by Kat Duff (Atria Books, 2014)

The Secrets of People Who Never Get Sick by Gene Stone (Workman Publishing, 2010)

Tomatoland by Barry Estabrook (Andrews McMeel Publishing, 2011)

Transcendent Sex by Jenny Wade (Gallery Books, 2004)

Documentaries

Cowspiracy (2014), directed by Kip Andersen and Keegan Kuhn

Fat, Sick & Nearly Dead (2011), directed by Joe Cross and Kurt Engfehr

Fed Up (2014), directed by Stephanie Soechtig

Food Inc. (2009), directed by Robert Kenner

Forks Over Knives (2011), directed by Lee Fulkerson

For More Information

Please visit: thehealthiestpeopleonearth.com

Recipe Index

Index

Acknowledgments

I offer heartfelt thanks to my agent, friend, and hero, William S. Thomas, who also served as front-line editor and drill sergeant on this project; to Bill LeBlond, another hero for sure, who offered genius advice on sharpening the book's focus; and to Harold Leo, another hero and a lifelong friend, who offered good advice on every aspect of this book.

I also want to thank Elisabeth Johnson Pastrama, my excellent second cousin and the most righteous vegetarian I know. She shared with me her DVD copy of the documentary *Forks Over Knives*, an inspiration to me then and now. My thanks also go to Kathryn Marie White Matheson, my awesome Aunt Kay, whose home has been the scene of many lively conversations about this book, often involving many other members of the extended Matheson family, including Cindy, Gary and Chris, Patti, Clint, Carol, and Shannon, Jim, Vicki and Krista, Mark and Adrienne, Rochelle, and Tim and Diana.

Finally, I give praise and thanks to the wonderful folks at BenBella Books, especially CEO and publisher Glenn Yeffeth, Adrienne Lang, Sarah Avinger, Alicia Kania, Rachel Phares, Heather Butterfield, Jessika Rieck, Vy Tran, Scott Calamar, and Karen Levy, who have transformed my manuscript into a book and have made me proud to be a part of their family.

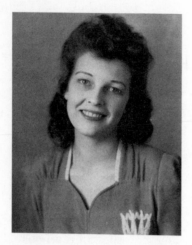

Dorothy Mae White Weeks,
mother of John Howard Weeks

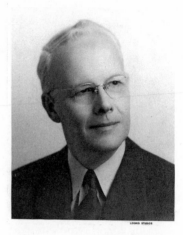

Herbert Clarence White, father
of Dorothy Mae White Weeks

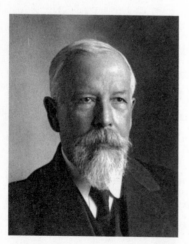

William Clarence White, father
of Herbert Clarence White

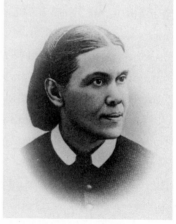

Ellen G. White, mother of
William Clarence White

About the Author

JOHN HOWARD WEEKS is a career journalist and longtime columnist for Southern California's largest newspaper group. He is author, co-author, or editor of six previous books (*Mojave Desert, Inland Empire, San Bernardino Bicentennial, Choice Words, Dream Weavers,* and *Window Beyond the World,* a novel). He has degrees in English literature from the University of California at Riverside and Birmingham University in England.

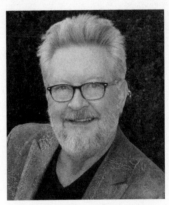

Photo by Mari Sarabia, Earhart Photography, San Bernardino, California

Except for one year in Europe, he has lived for more than fifty years in or near Loma Linda, California, the health-minded community established in 1905 by his great-great-grandmother, Ellen G. White, founder and prophet of the Seventh-day Adventist Church.